Survivor Stories

Speaking Out About Cancer

Survivor Stories

Speaking Out About Cancer

Edited By
Rod Schecter & Jessica Lynn Myers

Rivanna Health Publications
Charlottesville, VA

"Notes on My Dying" was first published in *Creative Nonfiction* 18, © 2001. "Juggling the Bones" first appeared in *Families, Systems & Health* (Winter, 2001, Vol. 19 No. 4).

ISBN 0-9676129-1-8

www.survivorstories.net

Printed in the United States of America

Cover image by Jessica Lynn Myers. Special thanks to Kemper Conwell from *Pixels* in Charlottesville, VA for help with graphic design.

Table of Contents

Forward

Before I started editing the *Prostate Forum*, my own experience with cancer had been piecemeal at best. Like most adults, I have lost enough relatives to speak about the *c-word* with the appropriate tinges of spite and acrimony in my voice: at age fourteen, I visited my paternal grandmother at the hospice, so disturbed by the sight of her—almost bald and a mere seventy-six pounds—that I never returned. I watched (or should I say listened second hand) from a distance as my aunt died of breast cancer while in her forties, and, as if it weren't enough, found myself racing home from college one spring semester to see my maternal grandmother just before she passed from the metastatic tumor that originated in her lungs. However, no matter how close cancer came, the images it inspired always seemed vague and abstract, replete with the gore and disfigurement of a horror film.

Even saying the word scared me in the same way, leaving scant room for hope in any statement compounded with the dreaded *c-word*. And sadly, without hope, even a horror film loses its potency, as the actors simply go through the motions before they ultimately meet their ends at the hand of the cruel antagonist lurking behind every corner. I realize this sounds glib, but to someone on the periphery of the disease what else can you say but "I'm glad it's not me," and withdraw from even thinking about what a cancer diagnosis means?

A dear friend of mine lost his father to colon cancer recently and the mere mention of what I do for a living turns his face pallid and grim. For him it is no longer an issue, a topic best not talked about in the light of day but in the sterile confines of an exam room.

But these are affectations gleaned from outside observation. Those inside the disease perceive things quite differently—know too well the vocabulary of "Cancer Speak" and learn to make the best of things. Even in this volume, Ruthann Robson's story *Palliative* mocks the alienating language of the medical community, hence reverting herself from research subject to person by redefining the language and making it her own. The same author, in another piece from this volume, clearly states her call to arms. "I am not your story," she shouts, in a language that speaks for a whole subset of people who are constantly made to feel like research by a medical industry fueled by its own inherent motivations.

The question becomes: if so many people are crying out, why are they being constantly ignored? It is too easy in our busy lives to shy away from cancer survivors—to chalk it all up to circumstance and go on with our healthy lives. Thus, we created this book to give a voice to cancer patients, to let their stories speak out clearly (not in hushed whispers), to let the world know they are survivors and still alive.

When my fiancé, Jessica, and I first moved to Charlottesville after a less than successful approach at living a bohemian lifestyle overseas, we stayed with her parents for several months. At the time, her father, Dr. Charles Myers (the renowned prostate oncologist), was suffering from prostate cancer and the debilitating side effects of aggressive radiation treatment. Talk about irony—a physician with the very same disease he himself had spent years studying. And he certainly knew about all available treatments—knew what to hope for, what the risks were, and exactly what his chances were. He knew, as he told me over the hushed breakfast table amidst his hot flashes and mood swings, that the best weapon any cancer patient had in his or her arsenal was the belief in the possibility of healing and a stubborn allegiance to hope. What I learned was that there was always some reason to hope and have since concluded that it is the infusion of even a glimmer of hope into a dark situation that defines what it means to survive.

In the following years, as I've worked on a variety of cancer publications and had the opportunity to teach therapeutic writing to patients and their partners at Free Union Institute seminars, I've became aware of more horror stories than I ever hoped to know about: intense pain, metastatic lesions, chemo side effects, and radiation proctitis. I also learned what a grim effect cancer treatment has on the human psyche. I was taken aback by how quickly a person can become their cancer, transformed until the growing cells are as much a part of their identity as the color of their hair. I've met activists in remission who still battle the awful disease that contaminated them despite the damage their obsession is doing to their careers, their marriages, their friendships. But there were others, the real survivors, the people who remained staunchly people (never succumbing to the label patient) who were courageous enough to tell their tales—each one as specific as a fingerprint—to tell the world that they were far from dead and would go out kicking and screaming if destiny was so inclined. The interesting thing was that these survivor stories were wrought with all the tension and conflict indicative of any satisfying story.

As literature students and aspiring novelists, Jess and I have often wondered what we could bring to a community where science is so dominant and hope that we've found that outlet in this small volume. It always seemed to me that, after every conflict, the stories are what remain to give credence to what was gained or lost. It is in the narrative form that so many people mourn and rejoice, and these survivor stories are as important to the teller as they are to the listener. In fact, I would say that it is essential to share our stories, no matter how painful they may be. We simply can't hide away from them. And providing a stage for those struggling with the indelible imprint cancer has left in their lives is as important as treating the survivor's body. The rationale: when the body aches the soul needs a place to mourn.

In each essay, our authors define what it means to survive: from a psychologist working in an oncology practice to a breast cancer survivor with two young daughters, these writers grapple with the impact cancer has had on their lives—the painful and the joyful—the moments when our vulnerability as human beings shines through to reveal something noble and achingly beautiful.

As Milton Ricketts notes in his essay, *Surviving The PC Jungle*, "Odd as it may seem, in some ways having cancer has improved my life . . . I no longer have good days and bad days; I just have good and better days."

The essays and stories in this book are meant to embody the experience of living with cancer, the ups and downs—the personal struggles and triumphs that some people face every day. In our normal lives we look to the future, complaining about the drive-though line, about the missed sales opportunity, about the annoying coworker, while a whole community of survivors trudge through percentages and experimental treatments, trying to buy themselves another tomorrow.

With that said, this book has the ability to affect not just the small sample of people for whom it was intended. *Survivor Stories* has the ability to teach us all that even in the darkest moments, there is always something to hope for.

—Rod Schecter   Aug. 2, 2003

Notes on My Dying

by Ruthann Robson

I believe in death with dignity, don't you?
At least in the abstract.
Grace. Nobility. Even beauty.
As abstract as that. As abstract as other people.

As abstract as characters in fiction.
"All anyone wants is a good death," I read. This is in a short story. It's a prize-winning story, a story about a nurse who is dying of cancer. She is graceful, noble and even beautiful.

I hate the story. I hate stories about people dying of cancer, no matter how graceful, noble or beautiful.

When I read the author's note, I learn that he is an administrator in the famous cancer center where I am enduring chemotherapy and the news that I am going to die very shortly.

This is what I say to his story: I do not want your good death.

This is what I say to his biography: You make your living off other people's deaths.

This is what I insist: I am not your story.

If I were constructing this as a story; with myself as the protagonist, I would be not only dignified; I would be brave and beautiful, courageous and kind, humorous and honorable.

I would enshrine myself in narrative.

But this cannot be a success because the elements of narrative are corrupted.

There is no beginning. The beginning is not diagnosis. The beginning is before that. Before the suspicions, before the reconstructed past when one began to feel this or that, before everything except a tiny cell that got twisted and frisky. The absence of the beginning is compounded by the middle collapsing into the past.

Everything is end.

Some endings are longer than others.

I am trying to act as if I have a future.

When I'm not too weak, I go to work. I go to the library and the post office. I go for walks. And when I am too weak, I go anyway. The worst that could happen to me is already happening.

I cannot pretend I am who I was a few months ago, so I pretend I am a fashion model. I am a Buddhist nun with a shaved head. I am anorexic. I have a lovely pallor. I have a noble beauty, a beautiful nobility.

I am not interested in fooling anyone except myself.

I call it survival.

I survived a dangerous adolescence.

In school, the sentiments of "Death Be Not Proud" belied its title. On the large and small screens, "Love Story" jerked tears, and the body bags and the immolated monks screamed for my attention. In the streets and bathrooms, needles in the arm and suicide sang their romantic dirges.

Not all of us made it.

When I made it to 21, 1 assumed I would live to 87.

Death was for the young. And the old.

At 26, I was hospitalized intermittently for six weeks with a strange malady that spiked my temperature to 107 degrees.

"You should be dead,' the doctor said, confirming my temperature.

"I'm not," I replied, thinking myself witty.

The year was 1984.

I was sure I had AIDS.

Instead, I was diagnosed with pesticide poisoning, contracted from the sugarcane fields where the migrant farm workers who were my clients worked.

A nurse told me I should be grateful for the advancement of antibiotics.

No one told me I should be irate about the development of agribusiness.

I knew I had almost died.

I thought I was cured.

There are those who argue that cancer is ancient, prevalent now only because other diseases have been cured and humans live longer, and unconnected to environmental degradation.

My body knows differently.

But who is there to blame? Industrialization? Capitalism? Corporate greed?

Anger is the second stage of dying in the classic work of Elisabeth Kübler-Ross. She notes that dying can cause a "usually dignified" person to act "furious:' but with a bit of tolerance by the caregivers, the patient's anger can be soothed. Dying people, above all, want to be heard.

I do not want to be heard.

I do not want to talk.

I want to live.

My first decision about dying is that I will die at home. I will have the control and comfort I would not have in a hospital. The winter sun will be weak but brilliant, sifting through my window, refracting through a prism I have had since I was young. Then the light will fade, leaving only a slat of brilliant pink. Twilight was once my favorite time of day.

My second decision about dying is that I won't. Like all my most outrageous ambitions, it first appears on my horizon as a question: What if? What if I refused to die? I am neither stupid nor naive and know that it isn't a simple matter of choice. Nevertheless, my aspiration persists.

The first stage of dying is denial. Ask anyone who has read Elisabeth Kübler-Ross. Or who has not.

Still, what if I refused to cooperate?

The manifestations of my resistance are illogical and small. I refuse Ensure, Ativan, a port, a wig. I refuse to talk to my oncologist, who warns me about depression. Depression, the fourth stage of dying, is the "preparatory grief that the terminally ill patient has to undergo in order to prepare himself for his final separation from this world."

If I were talking to her, I would tell her I am not depressed, though I may seem defeated, decimated.

I am simply deep.

I am inside myself so deeply the world is an abstraction. I cannot bridge the distance between myself and everyone else, including the ones I love most. The ones I said I loved more than life itself. Now, this is no longer true.

My death is only my own. No matter the connection, no matter the love. No matter that I came from the bodies of my parents or that my child came from my body or that my lover and I have joined as if we inhabit one body without boundaries. Each body lives separately. And dies separately. Perhaps I knew this before.

In the abstract.

I think about taking someone with me.

If I'm going to die anyway, shouldn't I kill someone? Shouldn't my death be useful? I scan my personal life but find no one evil enough to deserve to die. My passions are faded. I concentrate on the person I once hated most but cannot seem to despise him enough to deprive him of his narrow, miserable life.

Assassination is a possibility. I imagine buying a semi-automatic weapon. I have enough time for the license waiting period, to learn how to shoot, to do the legwork necessary to find a gap in the security. I think it would be relatively easy, since I'm not worried about getting caught. I would prefer not to die in prison, so I guess I'd kill myself as soon as my deed is done. I settle on a certain Supreme Court justice. But I find I don't care enough to kill him. Or even to think about it more than once.

Dying is lonely.

I am popular in my dying. People I have not heard from in several years call me.

"Is there anything you want to say to me?" she asks.

She is crying.

"My mother died of cancer," he says to me.

He must think this is an expression of empathy.

"You have always meant so much to me," she blurts.

She does not stumble over the past tense.

I never respond.

They must think I am being dignified.

Someone actually tells me this: "I really admire the way you are conducting yourself with such dignity," she says to me.

"I'm not."

"Well, it seems like that to us," she persists. She is a colleague and has always been comfortable speaking for everyone at work.

"That's not the way it seems to me." I prove I can still argue.

She smiles as if she thinks I am being modest.

I am not.

I am trying to be honest: I am all claws and sobs and vomit. I am small and getting smaller. I am bereft and bald. I am more tired than tired.

How could she not see that when she looks at me?

But she does see that. Despite the dignity, when she looks at me, she sees I am dying.

And when I look at her, I see my dying reflected back to me, a shiny, silvery object without form or function, an abyss of pity.

I am grateful for the people who do not pity me. Or at least who do not show their pity.

We have written letters for almost 20 years. When I write to tell her the news that I am dying, I ask her to try to write to me as she always has, to write to me about her life and what she is reading. She writes me every day. Every single, fucking day. Beautiful, exquisitely boring letters about her job or what she ate for breakfast or something she hopes will be amusing. I live for her letters.

We have written letters for eight years. I fudge the fact that I am dying but also ask her to keep writing to me as she always has. Her letters get longer. Pages and pages, which require extra postage, pages filled with assessments of novels, pages brimming with struggles about her own writing, pages of poetry. I reread every page until

I believe that I am strong enough to write back.

We have never written letters. She sends me a card. "Here's a second opinion: You're the greatest." It's in a package of gourmet food that once would have been appetizing.

We have lived together for more years than I can count. She was once my lover; now she is my caretaker. She tries not to cry in my presence. I am not so considerate.

She brings me books from the library when I can't get there myself. "Novels." I tell her, "from the New Fiction section." Sometimes she brings me the same book twice. Three times. Sometimes I recognize when this has happened.

Maybe I believe I can save myself through reading. Or at least escape. Or maybe it is that I have always read. Books were my first acquaintance with grace.

Although soon I stop reading fiction. I know she is screening the selections, but death penetrates the pages. Sometimes it is in the prize-winning story. Sometimes it is there casually and without warning. It seems there is always a convenient cancer death in the background somewhere, even if only in a character's memory.

In novels, they never recover.

Loss. Grieving. But life goes on.

I close the book and reach for the next one.

Soon I am requesting biographies. As if I have forgotten that the person in the biography is going to die. As if I didn't know somehow that Rachel Carson died at 57 of cancer. She hid it from the world, as if her dying were a recrimination of her work linking toxins with tumors in humans, an irrefutable rebuke that she was less than objective. Or perhaps she was trying to be dignified.

Desperation is not dignified.

Perhaps that is why Kubler-Ross does not name desperation as a stage. There is "bargaining," the third stage, but she gives it short shrift. She theorizes it as a belief in a reward for good behavior. She doesn't seem to understand the will to live.

It allows the decision to be strapped into a chair and have poison injected into my veins seem rational.

It propels me into the alleys of alternative healing, alternative theories, alternative alternatives. I visualize and vitaminize. I spread myself on the floor of an apartment in Chinatown so that a man can bruise my flesh as a way of clearing my meridians. I ingest herbs from different continents, animal parts pressed into pill form, teas that smell like mentholated piss.

I meditate.

There are those who argue that cancer is a message: Appreciate the beauty of each moment.

The moments most often invoked are populated with children. What could be more precious than the kiss of a toddler?

Other moments to be cherished occur in nature: oceans, sunsets, trees and their turning leaves.

Even a circumscribed life has its moments to be appreciated. The soft sheets of the bed, the taste of a strawberry, the flames in the fireplace.

Never mentioned are the moments in which I am managing to live. The moments, long and slow, during which I am dizzy and puking red on the bathroom floor, trying to appreciate the texture and temperature of the tile against my cheek. (How smooth! How cool!) The moments, as panic-filled as a fire, when I feel the chemical burn in my veins and watch the skin on my arm lose all its color. The moments, shallow and distant, when I try to think about anything other than what is happening to me.

Acceptance is the fifth and final stage of dying, according to Kübler-Ross. She warns that the harder the struggle to avoid the inevitable death, and the more denial, the more difficult it will be to reach acceptance with peace and dignity. In her examples, the patient wants to die, but the medical professionals believe it is better to prolong life.

This is not my experience.

My medical professionals are very accepting of my death. They proclaim it inevitable and do not deny or struggle. They do not seem to believe it is better to prolong my life. They are very noble.

Perhaps they read Kübler-Ross in medical school. Or perhaps

they're simply burnt out. Or they know the grim statistics for my rare cancer and see no reason why I should be in the smallest of minorities who might survive.

I loot the world for survival stories. Not the narratives of Himalayan treks or being lost at sea, but illness. The bookstore has an entire section on diseases and five shelves on cancer. I inspect every title, except the "prevention" ones, looking for possibilities. I buy a book by a Christian fundamentalist woman who attributes her survival to prayer and coffee enemas. I buy a book by a scientist who attributes his survival to vitamins. I buy books on healing by popular writers who intersperse their homilies with anecdotes of people given "six months to live" but who are alive 10 years later.

Possibilities.

I do not want nobility or beauty.

I do not want a good death.

I want possibility.

I am in my office, looking at the diplomas on my wall and sobbing over all that accomplishment, now utterly worthless. The skills I had mastered are the wrong skills for my situation. I know no medicine; my last biology class was in ninth grade. I can't even cope; my degrees are not in psychology or divinity. I learned how to think, how to read, how to argue.

My faith—in hard work, in intellectual pursuits, in books—has been misplaced. Nothing I know could save me. I want to rip my diplomas from the wall.

With dignity.

But I don't have the strength to carry a single book down the hall to the classroom. I can't stand up more than three and a half minutes. I no longer have the ability to assassinate that Supreme Court justice or to recall which one I had singled out as especially dastardly.

Still, I refuse to accept I am dying. I prefer denial, anger and even desperation.

When I can sit up, I spend hours at the computer, leaving no Website unturned. I become an expert in my rare type of cancer. A medical dictionary replaces my thesaurus.

I read books, articles, pamphlets. I have begun to eschew fiction. I want true stories of survival. I relish attacks on statistics and science.

I avoid all eulogies, all obituaries. I do not update my will or think about the existence of my property without me. I don't care what happens to those hundreds of letters, the ones I have written or the ones I have read. I don't worry about my office and its diplomas. I am not interested in any legacy.

I try to think. To argue.

There are those who argue that cancer is an infectious disease, like tuberculosis, because a gene-based disease would have been eliminated through natural selection. Cancer could be cured by the correct antibiotic.

I would like this to be true.

Now.

I had thought I had looked at death before. I had seen her dance with the ones I loved who have died. I had suffered my own flirtations. This time, though, death is gazing back. Not just a glance, but a full, seductive stare. As if we are in a bar and I am dressed in black leather, ready for adventure tinged with danger.

How alluring to be chosen.

This is what she whispers: I can follow her with grace and dignity. Or I can resist and it can get ugly. Either way, she will win, she promises me.

That is her story.

If she writes my story, I will be brave, beautiful and dignified. The word struggle will be used but with no incidents of sweating or cursing or thrashing. In her story, it will be as if I have fallen into a deep sleep.

As long as I am still able to write, this is my story: I resist the lure of dignity; I refuse to be graceful, beautiful and beloved. I am not going to sleep with her. I'm going home, alone.

Back to my books, my computer, my Australian herb and shark cartilage, my visualizations, meditations and bruised meridians. Back to my bedroom with the prism at twilight. Back to my office and its useless diplomas.

Back to my life.

we do not believe in ourselves until someone reveals that deep inside us something is valuable, worth listening to, worthy of our trust, sacred to our touch. once we believe in ourselves we can risk curiosity, wonder, spontaneous delight or any experience that reveals the human spirit.

—ee cummings

Calm Down, Little Cells

by Judith Boothby

My acupuncturist, Tally, says healing from cancer can be like digging a well when you are already thirsty. Even when it seems impossible, both cancer and thirsty-well-digging are feasible, if you have enough help.

It was early fall when Tally said, "Women with cancer who do counseling live longer."

"I have already done three years of counseling," I said. I could not imagine what else there was to learn.

"Women who do counseling live longer," Tally replied.

I noticed this conversation was mirroring a previous conversation we had had about me eating lettuce for breakfast. I now eat lettuce for breakfast.

So I called Tally's recommended counselor, Nan.

Nan asked me, "Why do you want to do counseling?"

I answered, "Panic wakes me every night. I don't know what to do."

"Have you worked with your breathing? It can help. People often breathe shallowly when anxious and it's calming to breathe deeper. More oxygen gets to the heart."

"Mostly I have been scared," I replied. "The doctors told me with certainty I needed to do a bone marrow transplant or I will die within five years. I went through chemotherapy seven years ago and was just starting to feel better. I don't want poison myself again."

She said, "I've just started to work with people dealing with cancer." I said, "Here I am."

A week later I showed up for my first appointment. Nan's yard had so many plants it was a safari getting up the steps to her house. Most of me felt safe with her from the start although it would have been hard to tell from seeing my tensed body. It took a long time for my nervous system to imagine safety.

In therapy Nan read to me from books about surviving and healing from cancer. I'd cry when I'd hear the word metastasis, or imagine leaving behind my child. Once she said, "Say it out loud; I am afraid to die."

So I said, "I'm afraid to die" in sobbing broken speech, and she leaned her forehead lightly against mine. Her touch felt good, and I felt her company with my grief. After crying, I was a little less afraid.

"The world offers black and white choices, like `Do you want to do chemotherapy or do you want to die?'" Nan told me. "I recommend creating a third way, your way. What this takes is strengthening your ability to stay present, especially when its hard to, so you can create or notice windows of opportunity." While listening I stared at the bouquet of yellow daisies next to her and thought about what she said.

My body hurt so much it provided me a wealth of opportunities to practice opening to unpleasant feelings. One day I had searing pain in my hip and pelvis and I curled up in a ball on the floor crying while Nan lightly rubbed the base of my neck. I felt supported by her gentle touch in a way that words couldn't reach me. At night, when I'd wake up terrified, I'd breathe and imagine Nan's presence and I could start calming myself down.

I am a chiropractor and during chiropractic school I was taught to view people with cancer as a malpractice risk and to refer them out of my office as soon as possible. Yet Nan invited me into her home. For two years, week after week, we'd walk past her parlor grand piano to the little therapy room. She'd introduce all of her lessons with the sentence, "Let's try an experiment." I have a much easier time showing up for the hard lessons when it feels like I have a choice.

"It takes stress off the nervous system to follow action with nurturance, then nothingness, before coming to clarity and taking the next action," Nan said. I was specializing in action, so this teaching helped me learn to stop for a moment when I finished a chore and let myself feel satisfied before letting go and deciding what to do next.

Through Nan's slow lesson on how to feel safe while I felt my terror, I learned how to get to my edge and create a new way. I appreciate why I came to this planet even more now and believe in turning towards and feeling all that is hard. I felt listened to, valued, and touched by Nan.

One day while I was watching the movie "Rachel's Daughters" with her I realized something else. We were watching nuclear explosions, poison being sprayed over food, and a lineup of one-breasted chests, when I started shaking. Nan was crying and she reached over and took my hand. While she held my hand, my fear of holocaust and dying of breast cancer diminished, yet another fear was unveiled.

I could not deny that I loved her. I suddenly knew that love is all we have to give each other. I needed sunglasses to look at this love I had for her. She had made it interesting to feel pain. How could I not love her after all the times she helped me down her front steps as my body rattled to hook up the old parts with the new ideas? How could I not love her as I watched her stop by the tall grass in her front lawn to feel the warm sun on her back?

But a worried part of my heart asked, "Does this love have to do with romance?" "No, no, no!" the rest of me shouted before my heart had even finished speaking. "How dare you even ask?" A little dent was left in that soft beating muscle of my heart where the question came from. I wondered if either of us was strong enough to withstand my asking the question, "What do I do with this love I feel for you?"

I was hoping to work through my confusion about love in therapy with Nan. However, our planet is polluted, and before I had much time to ponder the love word and separate it out from the mass media version used to sell products, my world suddenly changed again.

The memory is vivid in my mind. I'd brought the fish quilt I'd just finished for my son to show Nan. She laid it out on her living room floor next to the piano while she looked at every square. For the first time I said, "I am feeling better and I'm ready to celebrate."

She reached over with tears in her eyes, took my hand and said, "I have just been diagnosed with breast cancer."

There is only one thing worse than getting diagnosed with cancer and that is having someone you love get diagnosed with cancer.

Nan had a lumpectomy and soon returned back to work. A couple months later I asked her what she had chosen to do about the chemotherapy and radiation question. She said, "I chose not to do those things. I chose other things, even though I am not assured that my path would save my life. I do know that following my own path will give me my own life, which I very much want. It was helpful and supportive to me that you had jumped off that cliff in front of me!"

I said, "Oh."

The whole concept of cancer leaves me feeling like a little bird pushed out of the nest too soon. I noticed how I wanted that false sense of security knowing Nan was choosing the standard medical treatment, even though I had not chosen that option. The next week Nan told me she was quitting her work as a therapist.

Nan needed to be on her own path and I was heartbroken. If my therapy had ended more routinely I could have let go of that relationship, but this was cancer, a word that drives me to search for priorities, and then action. How could I let go of her when I thought she would be needing me? Nan said she couldn't imagine being daily friends with me. I suggested we could be awkward infrequent friends through the e-mail and she agreed to this.

Three years passed and my five-year skipping-the-bone-marrow-transplant anniversary came up. I became a living outcome statistic after having been given a zero percent chance of surviving. Now the medical researchers started contacting me. The letters said things like, "We noticed you are still alive and we suspect you used alternative treatments. What do you think was the most important part of your healing from cancer? Choose only one: diet, exercise or friends."

I called up the researcher and said, "Why don't you sit down and have a talk with me? After all, I was told with certainty I would be dead by now if I didn't do a bone marrow transplant."

The researcher responded casually, "Oh we don't do bone marrow transplants any more for the type of cancer you had. They didn't prove to be effective." I deeply wanted an apology from someone.

Before I had time to digest my rage I got a letter from another hospital. "If we hired alternative care providers would you come back?" I wondered how they were planning on mass producing the uniqueness of my health care providers. I wanted the system to embark on a journey of cooperation with alternative providers and with patients, as I try to do with my patients. I don't want medicine to co-opt alternative health care.

I got a third letter from another hospital. "We are studying breast implants and have you ever wanted one?" I sent back my opinion written in bold letters on the form.

You know I was told I would be dead by now and that the only way I could possibly stay alive would be to destroy my health with a bone marrow transplant. I managed to stay alive. Do you have any interest in this?

I got a letter back which effectively said, "We filed your letter and you can rest assured should we ever need the opinion of someone that has actually had cancer we will be sure to contact you." I wanted someone within the cancer business to start asking the important questions about medical care.

A year later, I ran into Nan at a rally to let our senator know a war with Iraq won't help. We are both healthy. It's been six years for me and close to four years for Nan.

I was not surprised to see Nan at this rally since our dominant cultures approach to both international disagreement and cancer are the same—war—obliterate anything that threatens us. We need to change this. We need to have a generous spirit and help work to transform these horrendous experiences into gentler lessons, little by little. Hold dear to your heart the option of acting from love and not fear. Most of us feel marginalized to some extent; love and trust yourself enough to have the strength to resist authority. Move toward a love for oneself and the world that affirms life, especially when facing death.

I believe it is love, the awkward kind, that repaired my heart and my nervous system and perhaps even saved my life. Even though I spent many tough moments learning that I could trust myself with love, there were no nasty side effects on my healthy parts.

From my experience with cancer I say: Do not be dried up by the thirst of the cancer epidemic. Open your heart and get brave enough to look at this cancer thing. Build many wells ahead of time. Grow softness and strength, before you are forced to, so you have resources if this crisis occurs to you or your loved ones. Face your demons instead of running away from them. This helps shift the balance of human thinking away from cutting, burning, and killing that which we fear. Love can affect the outcome.

Surviving The PC Jungle

by Milton Ricketts

The most frightening period of my life was when my wife, Carol, was diagnosed with breast cancer. The thought of her being in great pain or of my having to continue life without her was not acceptable. We immediately began doing our homework—studying the disease, investigating the various treatment options, and searching for the right doctors. Carol finally elected to have a breast removed and after the operation, her doctors felt that no further treatment was required. She recovered rapidly and we were relieved that all was well.

Our euphoria was rather short-lived because I stupidly skipped two annual physicals. When I finally had my physical, my PSA came in a tad high at 16.5 and the GP urged me to see an urologist as soon as possible. The urologist I selected had a great reputation, but I was a little skeptical because he had been one of my son's playmates, so I still envisioned him as a child. He convinced me that he had gained some maturity and wisdom in the intervening years and that he really was qualified to poke around inside me. Part of the poking was, of course, the biopsy. At a follow-up meeting with the doc, he informed me that I had failed Biopsy 101. I had prostate cancer.

The urologist explained that with a PSA of 16.5 and a Gleason Score of 9, I had a serious disease. (Now, there is a statement that will really get your attention.) He outlined eight or ten treatment options, but said two of them—surgery and watchful waiting—were not acceptable choices for me. Surgery was discarded because my disease was too advanced and I was too old. Watchful waiting was also not a consideration, because I had a very aggressive and fast-growing disease. Thus, without some form of treatment, I would have a short life expectancy. On the positive side, my health (other than the cancer itself) was excellent and most of my ancestors had lived to be almost 100.

Although I was unlucky enough to be diagnosed with advanced local prostate cancer, I was lucky enough to do it at the right time—

about a year after Dr. Charles Myers was diagnosed with prostate cancer and began writing about his progress in his monthly newsletter. My problems were quite similar to his, but I chose a slightly different path through his treatment decision tree because at age 70, I was somewhat older than he. Also, my aim was not necessarily to extend my life, but rather to have the best quality of life for the longest time. Hopefully, the treatment plan I chose, 3D conformal radiation and two years of hormone deprivation, will accomplish just that.

In its initial stage, prostate cancer doesn't hurt; that is, there is no physical pain, but it really does a job on emotions because of its unattractive long-term problems. Perhaps Carol and I were less affected in this respect than most couples because we had just dealt with her breast cancer. And when one gets to be our age, you begin to realize that much of your life is behind you. It would be nice to have many more years, but we are grateful for having lived long, interesting, and loving lives. On the other hand, I can appreciate how a younger man with a growing family would be devastated by the prospect of an early death by prostate cancer.

In the case of any serious medical problem its prudent to get a second opinion, but perhaps I overdid it. I insisted that the biopsy be re-evaluated by the super-pathologist at Johns Hopkins and I got three additional opinions on the diagnosis and treatment options. Because each medical discipline seems to prefer its own area of expertise as the preferred option, I contacted another urologist, a radiation oncologist, and a medical oncologist. By the time I sifted through all of the doctors' recommendations and all of the information that Carol and I amassed through reading and surfing the net, I was satisfied that I had chosen a reasonable course of treatment and had selected the right doctors.

Choosing the right treatment plan and the right doctors may be no more important than choosing the right exercise, nutrition, and supplement plans. I elected to follow world-class cyclist Lance Armstrong's approach to recovering from cancer. In his inspirational book *It's Not About the Bike*, Armstrong, describes how he used exercise, diet, and supplements along with a large dose of courage to beat cancer and to subsequently win the Tour de France. I was about 40 years older than Lance and not a world-class anything, but it seemed like a good idea to me because, except for the cancer, my health was quite robust.

The docs advised me that two years of hormone treatment (Lupron) might weaken my relatively strong bone structure, but that

I could mitigate the degradation by doing resistance training. By coincidence, I had been a highly competitive weight lifter in my younger days and had resumed lifting for fitness sake a couple of years before the prostate cancer diagnosis. The first step in doing what turned out to be an interesting study was to establish a strength baseline by recording my best efforts in a number of exercises, as well as recording my time and pulse rate on a three-mile jog. I stopped exercising during radiation and for three weeks thereafter. The idea was to not resume my exercise routine until three weeks after completing radiation, then begin resistance training three times a week for about an hour and fifteen minutes as well as jog, walk, or whatever for 45 minutes on the alternate three days. The initial test after resuming exercise indicated that I had lost about forty percent of my strength because of the effects of radiation and Lupron. Likewise, my aerobic effort had decreased about 50 percent. However, after 22 months, my upper body strength recovered to 80 percent, my lower body strength to 90 percent, and I could walk and jog a slow three miles. Some of the loss might be attributed to aging. It is interesting to note that during radiation and a couple of following weeks I lost 12 pounds, but as I got up to speed with exercising, I gained 16 pounds while my percent body fat remained constant at about 15 percent. My conclusion is that it is still possible to gain muscle when you are 73 years old, even if you are in prostate cancer therapy.

During the two years of hormone treatment I missed a few days at the gym because of an old shoulder injury, a few days because Lupron side effects hammered me too hard, and a few days when I just wasn't emotionally up to it. On many days a hard workout would consume most of my energy, so I was compelled to take a nap in the morning after the workout and another nap in the afternoon. Thus, I found that I was not an iron man like Lance Armstrong. None-the-less, I was still in better shape than most men my age. I had an annual physical performed by a new GP and when he called me to report the test results, he said, "If I had not met you, I would have thought I was looking at test results of a thirty year old woman."

It is possible that I over did the exercise thing or perhaps Lupron finally took its toll, because in the 23rd and 24th months of hormone depletion, I again lost strength and was barely able to exercise. Now that I am off the stuff and presumably regaining some testosterone, it will be interesting to see how much strength I will recover.

Explaining my diet is very simple—I follow Dr. Myers's guidelines very closely and I have learned to like it. On the other hand, I don't make a fetish of the diet. If a dinner hostess serves dishes that aren't on my diet list, I stay in the hostess' good graces by eating small portions and enjoying the opportunity to cheat a little. It is nice to give yourself a reward now and then.

My nutritional supplements have varied somewhat over the last couple of years, but the ones listed below have generally remained constant. I have caste out a few supplements that I thought were not helping and a few that peer-reviewed studies indicated were possibly detrimental.

As I said earlier, I selected a treatment plan that I thought would give me the best quality of life, but I knew that it wasn't going to be all honey and roses. Because the radiation field had to be broadened to include the first echelon of lymph nodes, the doc warned me I might have some problems with my colon and urinary tract. Sure enough, I developed radiation proctitis and had a considerable problem with my waterworks. Traveling any distance by any mode of transportation was out of the question for over a year and I still don't go anywhere without my "emergency" kit—baby wipes, toilet paper, extra underwear, and ibuprofen. After two years, both the front and rear plumbing systems are almost back to normal and my mobility has increased considerably, but I still can't fly unless the airline will guarantee me exclusive or immediate use of a potty.

Then there is the little matter of hot flashes—they aren't all that much fun. They were not too bad during the day, but they really zapped me at night. I believe I detected a correlation between increased sugar intake with increased frequency and intensity of hot flashes, but I wouldn't bet my remaining life on it. More important, I found the best way to alleviate hot flashes was with what we sailors call a crew fan. It is a small portable battery-operated fan that can be taken to bed with you, set on your desk, or walk around with if you wish. I have to confess that I no longer sleep with my wife and that she has been replaced by one of these neat little fans. The fans run about 400 hours on four D cells at low speed and a somewhat shorter time at high speed. Don't leave home without one.

When I first started hormone therapy, I wondered what all the fuss was about—it didn't seem to bother me. But by the end of two years I started looking for the truck that repeatedly ran over me. I was on four-month Lupron and found that it does not have a nice even delivery rate. The middle two or three weeks were a real kick in the head, so I gave myself some extra rest time.

Another vexing problem that I experienced with Lupron was

serious emotional dips and mild depression. Sometimes, for no reason that I understood, I would find tears rolling down my cheeks while at other times I would find myself in a blue funk for some imagined offense. The doc prescribed one of the new anti-depressants and I quickly found that the normal 20 mg dosage devastated me, but that I became almost human if I took only a 5 mg dose.

The most helpful thing a man with prostate cancer can have is an understanding partner, particularly if you are taking Lupron. You tend to be moody, emotional, apprehensive, forgetful, and sexless—a real bad combination that puts a strain on any relationship. My poor wife has an extra burden to bear because I am almost totally color-blind. Guess who has to determine if I have blood in my urine or stool? I think it was Robert Burns who said something about wishing to see ourselves as others see us. Well, we can't, but an understanding partner can act as an insightful mirror. Whenever I deviate too far from perfection, Carol has a nice way of guiding me back within acceptable limits.

At first I was reluctant to visit a prostate cancer support group. I imagined a bunch of sick old guys sitting around having a pity party. Was I ever wrong! They're a bunch of activists who're helping each other and promoting prostate cancer education. I soon found that boring my friends and relatives with my cancer problems and solutions was a quick way to alienate them. Then I found that talking with support group members who had "been there, done that" was not only comforting but highly useful in learning how to combat the cancer. After about a year of regular attendance, I now go less frequently, but I try not to miss meetings that feature top-notch speakers.

I am a little reluctant to write about sex because I don't remember much about it—Radiation and Lupron have effectively removed any trace of it from my mind. There is some chance that the ability and desire will return, but if it doesn't, so be it. We enjoyed a wonderful relationship for ever so many years, but no more than today's platonic activity. A big hug and a little kiss still sends shivers down my spine.

Odd as it may seem, in some ways having cancer has improved my life. I am much more aware of the needs and feelings of others. I have an urge to try to make life more pleasant for all those around me: family, friends, and strangers. Little things that used to annoy me now seem so insignificant. I really don't know why, but I now enjoy an inner peace that was never there before. As a result, I no longer have good days and bad days; I just have good days and better days.

Do I worry about the future? You bet, but I don't obsess about it. There is a high probability that the disease was systemic before I started treatment, but, after two and a half years, I'm doing great and think there is a possibility that I may have dodged the bullet. None-the-less, I have taken the precaution of setting up my estate so Carol will able to live comfortably if I'm no longer here. I have also seen to it that there will be something in the educational pot for the grand-children. I have accepted the fact that I am not immortal and that I have to die sometime. On the other hand, I don't relish the thought of having the disease metastasizing to the bone and causing great pain. All things considered—I' rather be run over by a truck.

Where am I now? My docs seem very pleased that hormone therapy has kept my PSA below 0.05 for 18 months and think it is time to see how I will do without it. By watching the PSA rise in the absence of Lupron, they will be able to judge how aggressively they must treat my cancer in the future. The best-case scenario will be remission. The worst-case scenario is that I will start chemotherapy or go into a trial. The hopeful scenario is that I will be able to keep the PSA within reasonable limits through intermittent hormone therapy. Whichever way it goes, I expect to be around to smell the roses for quite some time. My incentive is to be able to enjoy seeing my baby twin granddaughters grow into girlhood.

Juggling the Bones

by Deborha Derrickson Kossmannn

I've been thinking about death, and it seems to me that it is the disappearing that stumps people—how someone can be there, and then suddenly not be. At my niece Maddie's sixth birthday party, Steve the Magician was pulling a long rope of yellow and pink scarves from his shiny black hat. The younger children were stunned into amazement, but my oldest niece, Sarah, who is eight, was trying to figure out the trick. "Look, Aunt Debbie," she said, "This is where he puts it. And here," she pointed, "is where it must go afterwards." Sarah tried to make a straight line from what she saw at the beginning to where the trick ended. She wanted to be certain of what would happen next and believed she would eventually figure it out if she just looked long enough. Thinking about death reminds me of the magician and my nieces. Each time I try to figure out what I feel, another dazzling scarf disappears.

As a child, I encountered only sudden death. When I was seven, my orange cat attacked some baby rabbits. I found their small, shivering forms, ripped-off tails, and reddened flesh in the backyard nest. My mother brought them into the house and tried to feed them with an eyedropper, but they did not survive through the night. In the morning I went upstairs and found the baby rabbits sleeping and touched their chilled bodies. I don't remember burying them, but know we must have tenderly placed their soft bodies into a dark hole. My beloved grandfather had a heart attack when I was eleven and was taken away from our house in an ambulance in the middle of the night. He had walked me home from school that day and we'd read aloud together after dinner.

It wasn't until I was almost thirty that I was involved in a slow death. My grandmother was diagnosed with stomach cancer. For the last month of her life she lay in her hospital bed on the hospice floor of the nursing home where my mother worked. I was able to see how her stomach had become large from the cancer. In her last few weeks, it looked as if she were about to give birth at seventy-nine. Her bones became more delicate as the flesh disintegrated away from her body. Her small twigs of arms seemed as fragile as the skeleton of a bird's wing. My grandmother hoarsely asked me to give her sips of water through a straw to moisten her mouth. The morphine kept her quiet. I didn't move from the chair beside her bed. Everything was still except the light outside her window that grew grayer, then purple, and finally transformed into a deep blue as I sat with her during one of her last evenings. My grandmother was not a woman capable of much intimacy, but she and I had a special closeness since I was the oldest grandchild. When I was seven she taught me to play Scrabble and she supported me financially so I could study abroad in college. I am from a W.A.S.P. family: strong feelings aren't always spoken. Her death was peaceful, but between her and me, mostly wordless, and I wonder sometimes now if she had wanted to talk more about certain things, or if she had felt afraid.

Five years after my grandmother's death, a long-term therapy client whom I'd been seeing in my private practice was diagnosed with inflammatory breast cancer. I resumed seeing her twice a week during her treatments as I had in the past when she had experienced times of great stress. When she was first diagnosed, she longed for her own death; she'd been suicidal for years. But she fought her cancer so vigorously that she'd surprised even herself—shedding her hair, her bone marrow, her depression, and finally, turning her longing into a different kind of love. One day she gave me a tape of her favorite songs. The first and last songs on the tape were the same. A solitary voice repeated:

> There's another train
> There always is
> Maybe the next one is yours
> Get up and climb aboard
> There's another train.

I saw her on a Friday afternoon and, at the end of our session, she lingered in the hallway outside my office adjusting the scarf and baseball cap that covered her bald scalp. She moved slowly because her bones hurt from the injections. "Goodbye" she said, turning around twice to look at me from the hallway as if she were going to say something else. "I'll see you next time," I said, "Take care of yourself." The following Monday, several hours before our next session, she died during a surgical procedure. I cried for her. At her funeral, attended by hundreds of people, the priest said my client's life had turned around. She had mentioned having new friends as we worked together before the cancer, but only after the diagnosis did she really see the importance of her life. Only after her death did I fully see how much she had made of her time.

It has been five years since that client died and I now work part-time in an eight-physician oncology practice. People ask if it is hard to work with cancer; what I think they want to ask is whether it is difficult to look at death. What is it like to stare at its gaunt and tired face with clear eyes? But what happens in therapy sessions is rarely, if ever, about death. It's about hanging on, sometimes through the impossible: missing parts of a colon, a breast, the lymph nodes, a lung, and the ovaries. The body is filled with secrets that multiply until they are revealed and by then, they have already taken over.

What have I learned from working in the oncology practice? First, like Steve the Magician's tricks, life is constantly filled with surprises. Second, life is like the floor of the house you inhabit. You walk on it and take its sturdiness for granted. Usually, the floor is covered by rugs and furniture. But cancer moves everything and sometimes rearranges the clutter so that the bones of the house, unfinished floors, white walls, grief, and the things that have been lost are finally seen clearly.

As one of the nurses put it, "Some patients get to you more than others." I've worked in the practice long enough that some of my patients are in the process of dying, some have died, and many are still living well with cancer only in the background. In many cases, cancer is treated like chronic illness. It is managed. The oncologists, the nurses, the psychologists, and the office staff all live with it too. I try to stay still and present when the losses happen. But that nurse is right. Some of them get to you more.

Stan was one of my first patients in the oncology office. He had lung cancer. I started seeing him after his lung cancer recurred after a lung resection four years earlier. He still smoked. I was supposed to help him stop. I saw him weekly in the chemotherapy suite where we hung out in big, comfortable vinyl chairs. The tube came out of his port like a lifeline to the bags, the medicine coming in. Once we determined that cigarettes had been the most consistent relationship in his life since he was eleven or so, smoking cessation was off the agenda. He was willing to talk, but mostly he liked to joke with me. He didn't have much family. He had young adult children and some good friends, but he lived alone. Hours in the chemotherapy suite can drag by. Time was really all I had to give him. We'd sit together while the bag of his latest medicine dripped into his chest. After fifty minutes or so, a nurse would change his bag and it would be time for me to move on to the next patient. And then another week of life would go by before we'd see each other again.

During the pauses between sessions, Stan thought. We began talking about how when he was fourteen he nursed his mother while she died of cancer. He described rinsing a cool cloth and placing it over her forehead. He gave her a sip of water. He held her hand as she grew quiet. The cancer spread from her insides, somewhere from the place of his birth, through her bloated stomach. She died slowly and in pain. He looked away from me as he told this story. He did not talk about what might happen to him.

After we'd been meeting for a while, his oncologist added radiation sessions to the chemotherapy. "I'm tired," Stan said. He said it like he was referring to the radiation, but it wasn't just the radiation. When we explored what else made him tired, he admitted it was his life, specifically the life he was leading as a cancer patient.

A medical crisis was beginning. A friend brought him to the hospital. Stan was dehydrated, a wrinkled shrunken version of the man he'd been only a week before at his chemotherapy session.

He smiled weakly in the emergency room when I saw him. He joked, "I know, I know, I should be drinking. I shouldn't become a raisin." I joked back and told him his doctor would make him plump as a grape.

A month before the hospital visit I noticed that he had begun to have trouble retrieving words. He'd say the wrong things. He'd have to go looking for certain words or ask me. Then he'd tell me a story and repeat it. He'd forget what the oncologist told him at his weekly visit. In the emergency room, all of it was worse. I could follow the thread of his thought, but it tangled and heaped up over us as he tried to ask me again why he needed a brain MRI. The neuropsychologist tested him the next day, piling the colored cards of the Wisconsin Card Sort Test on the table in Stan's hospital room, asking him to remember four words: robin, carrot, lamp and car. He could only remember parrot, his brain wanting to make sense of the bird and the sound, the thought floating up from the hospital bed where he lay.

"When you see him in the hospital," the neuropsychologist said, "you will have to repeat. Repeat whatever you say to him again and again so that he can grasp it."

It turned out that the cancer gnawing at his lungs had widened and spread, a deadly flowering that grew into his brain across the frontal lobe near his eyes. The tumor made his brain tilt sideways and all his thoughts seemed to be pushed out. During the few days he was in the local hospital having diagnostic work-ups, he became more disoriented. He barely understood what was happening as I explained to him again the results of the tests. He knew there was something wrong, but it eluded him. It was like he was reaching his hand through the fog only to forget he had a hand. He was losing parts of himself, grasping that they were lost, and then losing that knowledge in the confused pauses. I offered him a drink of juice from the glass on his table. Then I repeated the phrase. After five days, he was transferred to another hospital for emergency brain surgery. Somehow he survived.

Six weeks later we were again sitting in our chairs in the chemotherapy suite. He was able to think and talk. Stan remembered very little from the time of the operation. He had agreed to use a cane to help with his balance, "like an old man," in his words.

"Look at my head," he kept joking as he touched his skull. "There's a soft spot." Then, his face serious, he'd say, "I don't want to die like that, not knowing what was happening."

There is a look I have begun to recognize from my experiences with my grandmother and my first cancer patient. This look is not part of the patient's physical features, but instead is a little like looking at the person through the wrong end of a telescope. It's like a distance begins to open up and I'm watching the patient travel away. I have learned this means it is time to bring up death more specifically. Not mortality, which everyone talks about when they are given the space to do so after being diagnosed, but the look that means death is coming. Six months after his brain surgery, I asked the oncologist for confirmation about Stan's condition.

"Runaway disease" was how the oncologist described it to me. He told me it was time for hospice and that he would be talking to Stan that day.

"How long?," I asked.

"Six weeks, maybe as long as four months depending on how he responds to the last medication," the oncologist said.

I met with Stan in an exam room after the oncologist talked with him. It was clear that he didn't understand that there was nothing left for him but palliative care. He didn't understand that he would be dead soon. In that moment I was having trouble imagining how it would be when he disappeared. I was afraid to say the "d" word to him, since I was grieving myself and didn't want this to interfere with his own ability to process what was happening. He was frail and tired. His skin was dry and folding over itself. I had known him two years and all I could think to do when it was clear that he didn't want to talk was to offer to call him later and check in. When I did call him, I realized Stan didn't understand what the oncologist had told him. "It's not time for hospice," he said, "I don't understand why it was suggested. And they didn't give me another appointment." I talked to the oncologist and made arrangements to visit Stan at his home located a few minutes away from the hospital.

On my way to his apartment, I rode the elevator to the parking garage. I felt tearful. I'd decided that perhaps this work would turn out to be too difficult. Maybe I was not cut out for it. I was too emotional to be a good clinician for cancer patients. Perhaps I had too many of my own issues about death and loss. A woman on the elevator saw my ID that says medical oncology.

She looked sad for a minute and then said, "Oh, that must be very hard, but the people you work with must really appreciate it."

I was too surprised to do much more than nod as I stepped off the elevator, suddenly comforted.

I drove to Stan's apartment. I had never told someone he was going to die. He gestured me in and I sat down across from him on the sofa. He offered me a soda, which I refused and a Lifesaver—yellow, bitter, sticky—which I took. My nose was a little plugged up from crying on the way over. Stan had "Jerry Springer" on, but now that I was there he turned down the sound so the TV audience silently gesticulated. A black-clad girl tramped across the stage wearing a red-lipped smirk out of which no words emerged. Telling Stan he was dying was the hardest thing I have ever done. I told him that he didn't have much time left now. I told him he needed to think about what he wanted for himself in this process—if he wanted to remain in his own apartment and not spend his final hours in a hospital. I repeated again that the doctor said there were no real treatment options now. I used the words dying and dead. During this moment I understood why the oncologists sometimes danced, bobbed around, looking for a rope, anything to throw out, anything.

"How long?" Stan asked me. "I want to know," he said, a little angry.

I was tempted to evade the question and put it back on the oncologist, but I didn't want to dodge or weave. I took a breath in the pause between us. I repeated what the oncologist had told me.

"We can't know for sure. It might be a few weeks or a few months."

We talked about the oral chemotherapy.

"My sugar pill," he sniffed, and I told him it might buy him a little more time depending on his response to it and would help keep him comfortable. But I then repeated that it was not about "beating the disease" any more. He said he felt hollow. We talked about where he had imagined being buried. We both had tears in our eyes as we crunched the end of our Lifesavers right down to their empty holes.

Outside his small apartment was a garden, once thriving but now filled with bushy weeds choking what he'd created over the past years.

"No energy this summer," he told me.

We'd spent a number of previous sessions talking about the garden in great detail: how he'd planted tulips along the border and how he'd had some trouble with the rosebush. The day I told him he was going to die we sat into the evening looking out on the growth in his yard. He was worried about his young adult children—worried they couldn't handle his death. He couldn't envision his own loss of them. It was the only time he really cried. Everywhere in the tiny apartment were pictures of their growing up, their art, even childhood toys he had saved.

We had a ginger ale after we talked. I poured it into icy glasses and he started smoking the cigarette which I was supposed to help him give up and we looked at each other. He told me he was glad I was there. I told him that I felt sad too. He asked me more about the hospice program. It was as if he could see that he was dying, but it still seemed far off down the road.

"When I get that bad," he said.

I pushed him gently: "You need to decide now, when you still have strength." We made an appointment for later in the week after the hospice nurse and social worker were scheduled to visit him.

The same week I told Stan he was dying, my cat became very sick. She'd not been doing well for a few months. After I'd changed her food for the fifth time, tried the special vet food, the baby food, she again vomited everywhere. Lethargically, she sat on the arm of the sofa like a small, emaciated gargoyle, not even following me around the house anymore. Then, after her steroid pill, she couldn't even eat her cat treat when she tried to chew it. I watched her suffer for another day, wishing she could tell me what she wanted, what would help. I called the vet and cried as I talked to the receptionist. The vet was very kind when we finally arrived in the late afternoon. The waiting area was filled with baying dogs. The cat rubbed against my hand as if she knew that nothingness would be next. She struggled with the vet, hating needles. Even at the end, life was strong and pushing against everything: her fur and bones and teeth. Shaved patches of hair drifted across the exam table. Afterwards, the vet wrapped her in a towel so we could bury her in the backyard under the peach tree.

I thought, "What if she's not really dead in there?"

I was spooked when I picked her up and wished for the old-fashioned rituals of death. The closing of the eyes. The last stroking of hair.

It was as incomprehensible to my cat, as it was to my cancer patients, as it was for my grandmother, and as it is for me. After we returned from the vet, the other cat and I walked around the kitchen. There was a big, quiet space where the dead cat once sat meowing. I felt a primitive fear. Perhaps my cancer patient felt the same fear as his breathing grew more labored.

A few weeks after the cat died, Stan and I had our last session. Hospice nurses came to the apartment and a neighbor and friend cared for him, knowing that he wanted to remain at home and not go back into the hospital. I helped him move up in his hospital bed so he could be more comfortable and felt his vertebra settle, felt his bones on top of each other smooth and barely covered with flesh. I put Chapstick on his lips and held his hand when we said goodbye.

Once my first cancer patient asked if I would miss her. After we explored it together—the usual, "Why is this important for you to know" that therapy is made of—I said I would and I did. I missed her and her and him and him. How could I not? How could I not care about these lives that have disappeared and yet haven't? What I know of her, I use to care about another. Then I help him, until all those relationships continue on and intertwine like the big roots of trees traveling underground. From that darkness something new begins as the leaves unfurl and bloom. It is probably all I've been able to figure out about death.

Two nights before Stan died, I dreamt I was a magician standing in an empty, dark room. I was juggling bones, big and white like long sticks. They were straight with no joints on either end of them. I kept their smooth dryness in the air. I was looking up to see them. I dropped them sometimes, but I picked them up and tried again, hoping that each time I'd be able to keep them in the air longer. The bones were heavier than I expected them to be. Their whiteness flashed up and over my head in a bright arc as I tossed them into the air again and again and again.

Dead Reckoning

by Bara Swain

I dodge a stainless steel medicine cart and a nurse's aide with sil-ver capped front teeth and sprint down the corridor. "Ma! Ma!" I cry, as I wrap myself around my mother in an uncharacteristic hot-dog roll embrace.

Ma peels me away.

"Hello, Jean," she calls over my bottled hair to her first-born. "Thank you for coming."

My sibling nods, eyes vacant, a Do Not Disturb sign etched on her brow. "We missed the connecting train," Jean says, "at Newark."

"I forgive you," says Ma. Pat pat pat.

Jean looks like me—my distant sister, more or less. Here is the more: more frightened, more dandruff, more corrugation in her boxy face.

"Do you want to go to the lounge, Ma?" I ask.

Ma claps her hands. "That's a grand idea!"

Jean balks. She screws her lips and—"But won't it be too crowd-ed?"—tugs a coffee-colored tress.

Here is the less: less accommodating, less bone density, less hair.

I squeeze my sister's skinny arm. "I think, Jean, we'll be more comfortable there."

Ma, dipping slightly, pilots her I.V. pole starboard. I man the bow, Jean takes the helm, and Ma breaks wind. Her pinched face softens and colors and –("Shhh!" I warn my sister) finally relaxes.

The visitor's lounge has two couches, six chairs, a round table, a toaster, a sink, and a black and white TV. It has two Wandering Jews. Five, if you include me and my sister and my mother.

Ma looks wistful.

"What are you thinking, Ma?" I ask.

A nurse with rolling thighs washes her hands and hums "Love Me Tender." Jean combs her hair.

"Do you want to play Scrabble, Ma?"

Ma tightens the sash on her striped hospital gown. "I want to live," she says.

"Well," I say, "can you play Scrabble and live at the same time?"

The doctor is late.

"He's detained," corrects the nurse.

"But do you expect him soon? My children are here—"

"Open wide."

"—and I want them to be present when—"

"Wider, please."

"NO!"

The chunky nurse appeals to my sister. "I need," she says, "your mother's full cooperation if she wants to get well. Do you want your mother to get well?"

Jean gasps. I grasp my sibling's three-inch wrist and draw her—"Uh huh"—to her feet. We flank our dazzling Ma.

Ma says: "I want to see the doctor."

"He's detained," says the nurse.

Jean trades in five letters. Ma reads the New York Times. I copy a number from a matchbook cover to my date book. If it's not my boss's cell phone—"Is it my turn already?" —then it must be Federal Express. Or my channel-surfing tarot card reader with the Schenectady accent and Seaman's furniture.

The nurse returns bearing gifts: a carton of juice, a pre-sliced English muffin, and a tub of Mazola. "Nathan!" she calls. "Heads up!"

Jean ducks. Ma jerks her I.V. pole with one hand and—"Watch it!" —shields my face with the other. The carbohydrate sails over-head, followed by the butter alternative and a husky laugh.

The nurse pitches the carton at our table—"Cheers!"—then sashays to the counter. "Nathan," she says, "you gotta be quicker than that! Or I won't share my lunch with you no more."

The receiving end wiggles his hips. "That don't matter to me, baby. Not so long as I get dessert."

"Somewhere," says Ma, "a village is missing an idiot."

The doctor nods. "And how are you feeling now?"

"Well," says Ma. "I'm still a little short of breath."

"And the pain?"

"Not as terrible."

"Anything else?"

"Well, I still haven't moved my bowels. But I suppose that's..."

"The tumor, yes."

"In my abdominal cavity."

"Yes."

Ma sucks her lower lip. "So the liver biopsy was...?"

"Positive."

Still composed: "Is that good, Doctor? Or is that bad."

Stock-still: "It's bad, I'm afraid."

"Why are you afraid, Doctor," my sister says. "Do you have a malignant tumor, too?"

"And I should call Aunt Anita and cousin Mathew. And the library. Write that down."

"But he says there are treatments, Ma."

"Do you think I should call Sebastian? His second wife is pregnant again. Carol or Kirsten or some biblical name."

"Christiana," says Jean.

"That's right. Write her name down, too."

"Ma, we need to get a second opinion."

"Ron can teach my calculus class. I don't know who they'll get for the Promotions Committee. I should call the Dean, too, and the Union, I suppose. And—oh! I need to call my accountant! Write it at the top."

Suddenly: "Ma! Ma!" I cry. "I don't want to live in this world without you!"

"Baby, baby, baby. Come here, baby."

I press my boxy face against my dazzling mother's frame. She runs her fingers through my yellow tendrils.

"Ma," I choke, "what am I going to do?"

"Just live your life, baby."

Weeping: "But who will keep me safe, Ma? Who will love me?"

My older sister reaches for me. Gently, gently, gently, she pries me from our mother.

"I will," says Jean. Pat pat pat.

Crisis & Transformation

By David M. Ross, LCSW

The Journey Begins

Life-threatening illness takes us rapidly, without warning, to a place of profound fear and deep soul searching. When illness is further complicated by a rapid series of disappointments, soul searching defers to the fear and fundamental struggle to survive. Such a chain of events propelled me into my "dark night of the soul" and was perhaps the bleakest period of my life. "Dark night of the soul," refers to an archetypal journey involving a psycho-spiritual death and rebirth; and it was through this experience that I was moved to heal beyond the physical, to heal those aspects of my life that blocked deep emotional connection to others.

By age fifty-seven, I had experienced a meaningful life. I parented two sons from early life through college and was gratified to see them develop into wonderful, loving, and capable young men. With a master's degree in Social Work, I had built a satisfying career that included a position as Vermont Director of Field Operations in Social Services and Child Welfare and a private clinical social work practice in Vermont and then in New Mexico.

Moving from New Mexico to San Diego in January 1997 marked another milestone. I was in a new relationship, pleased about living on the Coast, optimistic about work and had no physical complaints. I was dealing with licensing exams in Clinical Social Work and was approved to sit for the written and orals. I had passed the written while in New Mexico and spent the first three months of the move preparing for the orals and acclimating to my new life. Then within the next three months, I failed the exam, received a prostate cancer diagnosis, the relationship ended, my financial resources became severely strained, and I was forced to move in with friends.

These developments catapulted me into a major life crisis and my overwhelming fear led me to believe I could not overcome the obstacles. I began telling myself my situation was hopeless and remained in a state of crisis for several weeks. I felt I was losing all that I had worked for and would not make it to the other side. However, I did not isolate myself, but instead stayed in contact with family, friends, and colleagues who empathized with my feelings but challenged the logic of my extreme fears. I became aware that my negative "can't do" thinking was, in itself, a serious problem and consciously forced myself to claim a new mantra that I repeated day and night. Not long after, I was driving to work on the freeway repeating over and over with increasing conviction: "I can do this! I can do this!" A car passed and pulled in front; it had a personalized license plate that read "YOUCAN2." While I am typically skeptical about signs from God, the synchronicity of this event appeared to be such a direct response to my words that I felt surprisingly comforted and encouraged.

The Search for Meaning

The writings of Lawrence LeShan, Carol Pearson, and Jose Stevens were pivotal in my journey through this "dark night." Dr. LeShan spent thirty-five years researching and working with patients with cancer. He concluded that certain forms of psychotherapy do not work for cancer patients. These include psychoanalysis and any other therapy that focus on what is wrong with us, our weaknesses and our deficits. He maintains that to alter the progression of this disease, we must discover our unique talents and interests and release any blocks to their flow. When he shifted his focus from looking at what was wrong, to helping his patients find their right "fit," approximately fifty percent went into long-term remission, including those with metastatic cancer. His work was inspiring and led me to a self-evaluation process. I acknowledged that, in fact, I had found a "right fit" with my life's work, but also learned that my healing required a journey into my past to release self-deprecating belief systems.

Carol Pearson, Ph.D., states that the quest to find our selves, to find deep meaning in living, is a heroic journey. To grow and transform our lives we must experience a fall or a decent from feeling safe. To have our dream we need to face our fears, including our fear of death. In the end, we have to take full responsibility for our lives. And, as I experienced, the journey is not easy, the lessons are difficult, and the knowledge is hard won. Time is often spent in what feels like a wasteland in which suffering seems to have little, if any, value. Pearson asserts that if the seeker refuses to give up and continues to face the unknown, the reward is a new level of meaning often about the deeper nature of our being, the purpose of life and how we choose to use our time and talents. In a psychological sense, it is by facing our pain that we eventually come to experience joy, by facing our ignorance we gain wisdom, and through confronting our fear we come to freedom. Unwittingly, this was the time for me to face my pain, ignorance, and fear.

Pearson's writing, specifically her description of the "destroyer" archetype was especially helpful. However, when I was initially introduced to this stage by a colleague who had studied with Pearson, I freaked, thinking this must be about death. I then understood that the "destroyer" refers to both death and rebirth, and that death is about dying to a way of being that has ceased to honor who we are becoming. It is a shift of consciousness from fear to one of greater faith and sense of purpose beyond health, relationship, professional identity, and security. Cancer, the failed relationship, the threat to my professional identity, and the loss of financial security were the ingredients that initiated my journey into the "destroyer."

Jose Stevens, Ph.D., author, mentor, and colleague also significantly influenced my evolution through this crisis. Dr. Stevens helped me understand and address several areas of my emotional life, present and past, including self deprecation. He reassured me, against my skepticism, that the crisis would end, and that there was the potential for a spiritual, emotional, and physical healing and transformation. He writes: "Aside from exposure to toxic materials and grief over loss, battered self-esteem is perhaps the leading cause of cancer formation."

Healing the Body

Despite repeated medical advice to have immediate surgery, I decided to wait until I retook the licensing exam before beginning treatment. Three months following diagnosis, I passed the exam and started making decisions about medical treatment. I was in the process of making arrangements for surgery when, in my research, I located two prostate cancer support groups. One had been organized by patients and had such a strong reaction against surgery that it was difficult to separate fact from bias. The other had been established by Israel Barken, MD, a local urology oncologist. Dr. Barken's group focused on medical management and a partnership between medical provider and patient. I liked this approach because it was consistent with my knowledge of immune-enhancing behaviors and practices I had gained from professional experience with HIV+ individuals and groups. While a patient/doctor partnership is non-traditional and a stretch for some physicians, it requires the patient's active participation. This active involvement is empowering for the patient and thus good for health and well-being.

Through discussion in these groups, I decided to delay surgery until I could gather more information. I learned that there are no definitive answers when it comes to treatment and all procedures have potentially serious side effects. Initially I thought that, with sufficient information, I could make a reasoned and assured decision. However, with additional information, the choices became more complicated and I found myself moving from certainty to confusion about the many options: surgery, radiation, seed implantation, cryosurgery, hormonal therapy, or watchful waiting. I chose to initiate hormonal therapy to arrest the cancer's growth, giving me time for further evaluation. After months of investigation, I decided to pursue treatment with external beam radiation. Throughout the forty treatments, I continued to work full time, checking my endurance each day by running down the medical facility's two flights of stairs prior to each session and then up again afterward.

Healing The Spirit

Along with healing the physical aspects of this disease, I had become equally committed to healing emotionally and psychologically. My tendency to worry created stress and unhappiness and although following what I believed to be my life's purpose, I knew I needed to go deeper. To maximize my healing, I needed to release the deeper emotional blocks that continued to have a hold on me.

I was the fourth son born in a five year period to economically and emotionally overburdened parents. When I was five, my eight-year-old brother, Philip, was hit by a truck and killed. Years later, we continued to suffer this tragedy in a cloak of silence. The ensuing emotional deprivation and pain led me to feel overly responsible for others. I thought it was my fault when things went wrong and that I just wasn't good enough. This was the foundation for a life-long struggle with self-deprecation. My parents' conflicts became mine. I felt my mother's pain and sided with her against my father, who responded to me in kind. As I aligned with my mother, the relationship with my father became more painful. Throughout my youth, emotional coldness, criticism, and anger characterized my relationship with him.

The correlation between the father/son relationship and cancer was the subject of a study of 11,000 male medical students at John Hopkins University Medical School in the 1940's and published in 1991 in: Cancer Detection and Prevention. The participants completed a "closeness to parents scale" questionnaire and the subjects still continue to be followed. The findings are striking; the best predictor of cancer risk years later is a negative father/son relationship. The significance of this predictor has not changed with time and is not explained by other factors like smoking or drinking.

To heal the early relationship wounds, I had to recognize, acknowledge, and release my feelings of self-deprecation as well as the impact of my painful relationship with my father. With the support and guidance of my therapist, I began to release these layers of childhood trauma and with them, my feelings of powerlessness, victimization, and fear, and, as I learned to recognize unhealthy relationship patterns, I allowed certain people to move out of my life. I became aware that by holding resentment I was, in effect, draining myself of energy needed to support my immune system and healing. With deeper reflection and insight, I began to understand these experiences in a different way. I started to see that the people whom I believed had hurt me were also instrumental in my personal drive to grow, change, and respect myself more deeply. This process of reframing and recasting events from negative to neutral or positive, was another significant turning point in my healing. I was able to reach acceptance and compassion toward my parents and others knowing they had done their best.

The Gift

As the unfolding continued, I began to understand that my work with people with HIV and AIDS, as well as my personal experience with cancer and subsequent inner journey and insights, could be combined to help others learn about themselves, about the mind-body connection, and ways to support and enhance health and immunity. Thus, in the summer of 1999, I submitted a proposal to the Prostate Cancer Research and Education Foundation to support a seven-week psychoeducational group at the Wellness Community in San Diego. The group would focus on caring for our bodies, caring for and honoring our emotions and feelings, caring for our spirit, and doing what we love.

The proposal was approved in September and in the following two years the Prostate Cancer Research and Education Foundation and the Wellness Community co-sponsored six groups for a total of sixty men ranging in age from 50 to 75. The mind-body approach emphasizes the importance of viewing this disease as chronic rather than acute and on dispelling the fear-based belief that prostate cancer is a terminal diagnosis. The men learned about the connection between the mind, body, and emotions, as well as how thoughts affect feelings, and, thus, feelings affect the immune system. Each night included meditation and healing visualizations. We explored the nature and impact of stress, early life experiences, intimacy, potency, emotional vulnerability, and the concept of "doing" vs. "being," and "wants" vs. "shoulds." Resentments and hurts were examined along with the importance of forgiveness and acceptance. Finally, we explored the significance and value of living fully in the present to pursue our life's purpose.

Before and after group sessions, the men discussed typical subjects such as sports and world affairs, but once in session, they allowed a deeper level of personal sharing that included self-exploration, self-disclosure, and soul searching. They often spoke of how surprisingly safe they felt with each other despite an initial nervousness. For many, this was the first experience in a male environment that was non-competitive, supportive, and encouraged bonding. One member, for example, disclosed that he'd never had a close male friend and always felt the absence of this. He credited the members of the group for meeting this need. Another likened his group experience to the deep connection he felt with those he fought side by side with in Vietnam. Given the opportunity of a safe, caring, structured environment, the group members were eager to share and be open to others with similar concerns.

Looking Back

More personally, prostate cancer, a failed exam, a disappointing relationship, and threatened finances were the catalyst spurring my "dark night." Yet these were also the ingredients that served as a wake-up call, facilitating my most profound growth experience. Many times I wanted to stop, retreat, and give up, but, with support and persistence, I slowly recognized the light in front of me. Now, as I reflect on these last several years, I can see that there has been a deep shift in my life that would not have occurred without the introspection and changes that cancer forced. Five years post-diagnosis, my PSA (prostate specific antigen) continues at a near undetectable level with no further medical intervention. The urologist expresses cautious optimism about a cure. The pain of the failed relationship has been replaced by greater emotional depth in all my relationships. My professional life is deeply satisfying as I facilitate a prostate cancer support group while continuing my clinical practice. In the end, cancer, paradoxically, helped me become more aware of and connected to myself, to others, and to those aspects of life that give meaning as well as an ever-deepening appreciation and passion for living.

Epilogue

My decision to write an article of such personal nature came from several fronts. As a psychotherapist I understand the value of sharing our journey, and of the healing that comes from speaking from the heart and speaking our truth. Few experiences cause greater emotional discomfort than a prostate cancer diagnosis and there is too much silence about prostate cancer in general. This is in part because the word "cancer," has been synonymous with death, and because patients and families are uncomfortable talking openly about cancer, about death, about bodily functions such as incontinence, and about sexual potency. This silence keeps us less informed, more vulnerable, and at greater risk of poorly considered treatment decisions.

In this culture, men struggle with expressing feelings of fear and vulnerability.

The stereotype of the "real man": tough, unflappable, nerves of steel is unfortunately alive, especially among older men who grew up in the "John Wayne" era. And in some ways, this icon of what it means to be a man may be doing as much harm as the disease itself. Generally, the initial reaction to a diagnosis of cancer is something like: "What can I do to get this out of my body?" and "How much longer do I have to live?" In this crisis state it is natural to concentrate attention on the physical, on ridding ourselves of the cancer. While this may give some feeling of control, the feeling is generally short lived. Treatments are often of limited success with troubling side effects such as impotency and incontinence. Unfortunately, because of the fear engendered in the initial diagnosis, we tend initially to minimize these considerations and later regret not taking enough time. In fact, more often than not, sufficient time is not taken and the medical treatment is not adequately weighted in light of its full impact on the whole person.

The general trend in our culture is to put our health care, including treatment, in the hands of the physician. However, with prostate cancer there are many treatment options, and it behooves the patient to become an informed consumer and to take responsibility for the final decision. It is important to come to terms with the fact that there is seldom one "correct" answer and all treatments have potentially serious side effects.

In fact, given our current understanding about the treatment of this disease, all other medical interventions need to be carefully considered. I urge patients and loved ones to utilize the help of qualified therapists and cancer support groups, and encourage men to become informed consumers and equal partners with their health care providers.

In the end, the crisis of prostate cancer and cancer in general can be a vehicle to achieve greater quality of life. As an elder in the cancer community, I hope those who come to face similar struggles will benefit from sharing my experience.

Owls

by Kathryn Kerr

It was late winter, Friday night. Tom, my husband, had gone to bed. Nancy, my older daughter, was reading. I was sorting through junk mail, while our little one, Sarah, was constructing something with crayons, scissors, tape, and my discarded paper. We were all quiet. The first call came faintly, but we fell as silent and motionless as small creatures in the dark, exchanging glances that said "You heard it, too!"

Another series of hoots held us. Then Sarah broke the silence. "Who cooks for you? Who cooks for you two?" She was pleased with her recognition of owl talk.

I whispered, yes, it was an owl, but barred owls sing "who cooks for you" and this was another kind of owl. "Barn owl?" Nancy asked, hopefully, perhaps, remembering the barn owl that lived on her friend's farm when she was small. One summer night we had sat on her friend's family's porch swing listening to the barn owls. No, I was sure it wasn't a barn owl.

Now it called again, closer. HOO hoo-hoo HOO HOO! We were silent until it called again.

"Can you repeat that music?" I asked Nancy. "One—two-and three—four" she answered in the same pitch. Then she seemed embarrassed, shrugged, and said that's what her band teacher would say.

It called again. Sarah had come to lean against me and peer out the dark windows, sucking her thumb. "One and-two three four?" I asked Nancy, not even attempting to match the musical pitch of the notes.

"Whatever." She shrugged, trying to seem cool, her eyes betraying her excitement. "O-o-o-w-w-w-l-l !" said Sarah, stretching the syllable into an owl's call, excitement spread all over her face.

But neither of them could have been more delighted than I. It had been about twenty years since I'd heard that call clearly, but I thought I knew it, still. I got the bird book and turned to the owls, reading their calls. Yes! I was certain it was a great horned owl! I showed the picture to the girls. Our owl called a few more times. We sat looking at the book, listening.

"What does he want?" Sarah asked?

"A girlfriend," I answered, "or a boyfriend. Another owl to make a nest with and raise baby owls."

Nancy, edging into adolescence, liked that idea. The calls had moved further away. I read the text aloud to them. ". . . prominent widely spaced ear tufts; yellow eyes. . . . sonorous, far-carrying hoots. . . .largest of American "eared" owls. . . .one of the first birds to nest. . . ."

"Is he big?" asked Sarah.

"About thirty inches tall," I said. "Look, Sarah, he is this big on you." I put my hand a few inches below her chin. Her mouth fell open. "But he doesn't weigh as much as you do. But a bird that big has to have big wings to fly, much wider than your arms." I stretched her arms out, then my own. "His wings are almost as wide as my arms." She was impressed.

"And they fly silently, Nancy informed her. "So then can catch things. Those big wings go silently through the woods because their feathers are soft."

Sarah was uncharacteristically still.

After the children are in bed I looked at the bird book, and sang that song in my mind. HOO hoo-hoo HOO HOO! Who who-who WHO WHO? Now, I'm a cancer survivor: two years ago I found out I had breast cancer. It had been a little over a year since I finished the treatments. I looked for omens that indicated I would raise these children. I thought that owl didn't call my name. In a beautiful novel I Heard the Owl Call My Name, a dying young priest is sent to live with Pacific Coast Indians who help him as much as he helps them. Part of that story turns on the legend that an owl will call your name if your death is near. This owl was questioning. I'm certain he didn't call my name.

When I got up the next morning, Nancy was still sleeping. Sarah was standing up in her high chair telling Tom about the owl who was this high on her (hand beneath the chin) and whose wings were wider than she could reach (she demonstrated), who flew very quietly so he could catch things to eat, whose feathers were soft. Tom was impressed by her knowledge. He steadied her with one hand, and then looked at me with questions in his eyes.

I nod my agreement.

I think I can raise these children.

Lucknow Woman

By Diana Marquise Raab

There is no breast cancer in my family. No cancer of any kind.
Except for mine, that is.

The bad news was bestowed on me last year. Before I had time
to accept what was happening to my body, I was lying on an operating room table in a strange city more than three thousand miles away
from home, having a mastectomy and reconstruction.

Why me?

No one could explain why I was diagnosed with breast cancer at
the age of forty-eight. Back in 1983, I can still recall making the
decision to breast-feed all three of my children. The literature
promised this was the best insurance against breast cancer.

My first-born, Rachel, arrived prematurely and she barely had
the energy to nurse. Within moments at the breast, she'd fall asleep.
Then I'd resort to this archaic pumping machine, feeling like my next
word should be moo, while suctioning my inflated breasts into these
plastic bottles, later to be fed to my daughter by some tight-lipped
nurse in the "preemie nursery." Rachel, I thought, would suck up all
those healthy immunoglobulins and my lymphatics would be stirred
up and stimulated so breast cancer would never, ever enter my life.

Why didn't I just give her formula? Wouldn't it have been so
much easier? I thought it would be healthier for both of us—physi-
cally and psychologically. All that bonding time. Maybe that was the
problem with my relationship with my own mother. She never nursed
me.

And then the studies. What about the latest one which has everyone in an uproar?

They say that only about five percent of new breast cancer cases
are hereditary. The rest are supposedly due to environmental causes.
Okay, this means we should stop eating and breathing. A few months
ago I read in the New York Times that the area where I was raised in

the fifties and sixties on Long Island has a higher incidence of breast cancer.

They think it might have something to do with the electrical lines. So cancer is blamed on modem technology. We're damned if we do and damned if we don't.

My father, who died twelve years ago used to say, "When your time is up, it's up." On his death bed, as he choked up secretions as a result of forty years of smoking, he said, "I've come to an end."

"Why do you think that, Dad?"

"Well, after you've survived the Holocaust and seen millions of people starved to death or slaughtered, you can't help to think that. I came out alive; I feel it would be greedy to ask for another chance to live. Gotta give someone else a chance."

"But Dad, don't leave us now," I said, looking around the hospital room at his three grandchildren, all under the age of ten.

As I glanced into his wet eyes, I saw that he had had enough. He had told me once that the only things keeping him alive were his grandchildren and me, but he couldn't hold on any more. A large part of him wanted to give up, and so that night he took his last breath. How astute he was to have called us to his bedside. We flew across the country to be there. Only moments before we handed him tissues to fill up with globs of sputum. I'd combed his hair and given him a back rub. Truly, I think what really made him surrender was seeing his own face in the bathroom mirror. "I almost fainted," he told me only hours before he died. "I looked like those people in the camps at Dachau. There was nothing left of me."

By the time I turned thirty-five, medical specialists started endorsing bi-annual mammograms. Five years later they'd started recommending one a year. I was an obedient patient and did as they said. Each year, I was singled out and they had me return to the hospital's x-ray department for additional views. "They're suspicious and want to make sure," the receptionist recited.

So I trekked back to the hospital and sat in a waiting room that smelled like a cross between hospital disinfectant and perspiring orderlies. The tables in the room were filled with shriveled and torn up women's magazines, harboring the same fearful topics with different headlines. The following week, they called to say that everything was okay. For seven years in a row I performed that ritual.

The May 2001 mammogram was different. I was called back in for repeat films and subsequently an ultrasound. During the ultrasound, while still staring at the computer screen in the closet-size room, the technician said, "Wait a minute," as she flung open the push door and stormed out.

The door closed by itself. I lay there quizzically, half-exposed. I looked around at the barren walls. It was dark and I was alone.

"What the hell was going on? Why didn't she tell me where she was going?" My eyes flooded and began burning from the globs of mascara I'd applied that morning. (For whom? The radiologist?)

Five minutes later, although it seemed more like ninety, in walked a middle-aged man wearing John Lennon glasses.

"Hi, I'm Dr. Schmo, the chief radiologist here."

"Hi, Dr. Schmo. What's going on? Why isn't anyone talking to me?"

"We're concerned. Give me a moment."

He sat down in the swivel chair facing the computer; his eyes scrolled the screen and then he looked back at me.

"You've got some calcifications. Can you see?"

"No."

"Well, these calcifications weren't here last year," he said.

Through my peripheral vision I saw him pointing to the screen with his pen.

"I'd recommend a needle biopsy," he added coldly. John Lennon was warmer than that. The radiologist's personality didn't match his looks.

"Shit," I blurted out as the room began spinning and I felt myself slip to the edge of the examination table.

"Are you all right?" he asked inanely.

"No. Would you be?" As a nurse, I felt I had the liberty to be blunt with someone exhibiting such terrible bedside manner.

"Why don't you get dressed?"

"I'm dizzy. Is that all you want to tell me?"

"Yes, in fact. You should call your doctor in the morning; he'll have all your results." The technician applied a cold compress to my forehead and the radiologist walked out.

I dragged my feet to the car and went through ten tissues from the flowered tissue box that had sat unused for months in the back seat. Finally, my voice became stable enough to phone my husband at work.

The following week I hopped cities to Dallas and was being prepped for a needle biopsy set up by a radiologist friend in Orlando.

While waiting for the team to arrive, I lay on the table writing my obituary. No one in my family could write, so I thought I'd help them out. That's the type of person I am. Always helping people out. That's my problem. At least that's what Louise Hay says in her book, *You Can Heal Your Life*. Breast cancer victims are often busy helping others before they help themselves. My daughter had just graduated from an emotional-growth school in Utah; we sent her there eight months earlier because she'd started hanging out with a bad crowd in an Orlando public school. We had no choice, and now we can say that it was the best decision of our life. To celebrate her graduation, all five of us took an extraordinary holiday to Hawaii. And now this? Where is the justice? Will I ever be able to take a deep breath again? Who's got it out for me?

I suffered every day of the eight months she was away. We had been more connected than a baby to an umbilical cord. I cried every night and wrote to her every other day, and spoke to her counselor weekly. Her changes were gradual, but hopeful. "Compared to others here, she's in good shape," they told me.

"What, are you kidding? She was catatonic before we sent her to you."

"Well, we've got kids here who've cut their wrists, jumped off buildings, were found comatose on the streets from drug overdose, beaten by their parents, and selling drugs illegally. Believe me she's in good shape."

I'd hang up and try to act thankful that her therapist even spent time speaking to me. But, while lying on the table awaiting a biopsy, I was far from thankful. I was pissed off. I had so many productive things to do with my life, so many books I wanted to read and write, so many people I wanted to love.

The radiologist told me the biopsy confirmed widespread DCIS (ductal carcinoma in situ).

"This is pre-cancer. It's very early. These calcifications can turn into a tumor. As a matter of fact, most tumors begin this way. If you'd waited, things would have been much worse. You got here in good time."

DUH.

The radiologist placed his arm around me. "I'm sorry," he said, as if my death certificate was already written. Glad I'd taken the time to write my obituary.

"So, what's my prognosis?"

"Good. It's good, but chances are you'll need surgery."

I remained cognizant, but silent.

"Like what kind of surgery? Don't pussyfoot around with me, I'm a nurse."

"It depends. You need to see a surgeon. He might recommend a modified mastectomy or lumpectomy. Probably the former."

"Would you be so straight forward if I were your wife?"

He offered a half smile—half rye bread, half pumpernickel. I wanted all the information and none of the information. I couldn't decide.

My husband and I returned to Orlando. I had mixed feelings about what was happening. My older self said that having cancer was taboo and that you didn't speak about it if you had it. People would start moving away from you. My young self said that speaking to everyone offers comfort and may help provide answers. I became someone I was not, and spoke to anyone who would listen. I was not going to hop up onto the operating room table and get chopped up.

I called my urologist, who over the years had become a friend. His wife had died of breast cancer the year before. He was a sensitive man and I trusted him. They had three children, much younger than mine.

"Go see Dr. M., a great oncologist," he said, without hesitation.

I marched into Dr. M.'s office and sat in the waiting room with a slew of seniors grasping onto canes and walkers of various sizes and shapes. Weren't you supposed to be old when you got cancer? Gosh, did I feel out of place. I thought about the breast cancer walk-a-thons I'd participated in, and all those women wearing wigs. Was I going to lose my thick head of hair, the first thing my boyfriends complimented when I was a teenager, after telling me they liked my green cat eyes. I went to the co-ed bathroom and pulled my hair back. Gosh, I looked crappy bald.

"Diana, if I were you, or if you were my wife, I'd suggest heading out to Los Angeles to see Dr. Mel Silverstein. He's a world expert on DCIS. I've seen him present at numerous conferences. He is conservative, yet sensitive. I trust he will tell you like it is. I can have my secretary set up an appointment for you," said Dr. M.

"I'm there," I said. "L.A. must have great doctors. What do Florida doctors know about breast cancer in a forty-eight year old woman? Don't they just know about senior citizens with breast cancer and the rest of them down here with some sort of skin cancer? Forgive me for generalizing, but I had no time to waste.

Dr. Silverstein agreed to see me the following week. The tall and sleek gray-haired breast surgeon looked as if he'd seen it all. I'd trust my life, my family, and my guts with that guy. Something about him exuded confidence. Was it his handshake? Was it the fact that he took me into his busy office right away? Was it his demeanor? Did it matter? It was his entire package. I was willing to fly across the country again to call him my surgeon.

"We know you have DCIS, but I will not know to what extent until I do a surgical biopsy. I'll ask my nurse about any OR openings. Can you hang around one more day?"

I nodded. "Absolutely. I want to get this all taken care of."

I loved this guy and didn't even know him. He was sensible and sensitive. I could just tell.

"My nurse Connie says we can do it in the morning. Be here by eight."

I gave him a soldier's salute. I was happy and petrified at the same time. Leaving the office I entered the sterile hallway with the gift shop across the way. The window featured wigs and T-shirts supporting breast cancer. I would have preferred a bar. A glass of chardonnay would have looked good pasted on my psyche. I got that jittery nervous feeling I used to get as a teenager when I craved a cigarette. I felt angry and defiant. A cigarette? That would be crazy. There was a chance I had cancer.

I gave the valet kid my ticket and slipped into my rented convertible. The top was definitely coming down. It didn't bother me that I'd forgotten to tip him. I drove in the direction of my hotel. The radio blasted rock and roll music, as I flipped back and forth from it to silence. I couldn't decide what would feel better beating at my brain, silence or rock and roll.

My thoughts skirted back to my father who, at the age of seventy, died of congestive heart failure. They told him he'd smoked too many cigarettes. He'd have a fit if he knew what I was going through. For sure, he'd hop on the next plane out of New York, just to spend the evening with me. I thought about my kids and husband, and wondered how they would survive without me. Even as teenagers they needed me. I posed many questions, but was void of answers.

At the Ritz Carlton they stiffly opened my car door and welcomed me back. I wasn't in the mood for politeness. Just park my damn car. At four o'clock in the afternoon I made my way to the bar for a drink—two drinks with a temptation for a third. Did these suave guys looking at me know that I have breast cancer? Would they still give me those seductive glances if they knew? I felt like testing them. NOT.

I returned to my room and removed my shirt. I stood in front of the bathroom mirror, raising my hands over my head like they did when giving me my breast exam. There was no dimpling. My boobs hung low, like they're supposed to after bearing and nursing three children. The areolas were stretched into an oval shape, but it didn't matter, my husband loved me anyhow. They looked normal. How could something as creepy as cancer be in there? I turned around and looked at my back. Not a bad body for a forty-something year old. I glanced again at my boobs. I shivered and got dressed.

That night I gulped down a sleeping pill to fall asleep. After waking up from the biopsy the following day Dr. Silverstein told me he'd call me in Orlando when he received the results. "Don't worry about flying home," he said, "Just take some extra bandages. You'll be fine."

He and his nurse hugged me and told me not to worry. Simultaneously they both said, "You're in good hands." I thought about what little effort that gesture took, and how calm it made me feel to have someone hold me at that moment.

I thought about the importance of little things in life.

That afternoon the flight attendants bothered me. I resented how healthy they looked and how I didn't even know if this was my last flight, ever. I loved flying, traveling and seeing different parts of the country, having new places, new experiences to write about.

The trip to Hawaii two months earlier had been awesome. Something about eating outside and living without air conditioning enticed me. I loved the way there were flowers everywhere. Down at the tennis courts they had pink bougainvillea floating in the ice-water pitchers at the courtside tables.

Part of me wanted to savor the experience of flying, yet another part of me wanted to ignore it. The people all around me knew nothing about the road I was headed down. For a split second I realized I didn't know anything about their road, either. How do we know who is healthy? It's not written on our foreheads. I felt anger creep into my soul. I became irate and impatient with anyone who crossed my path. How dare I be bestowed with cancer? I had too many losses in my life. When I was ten years old I found my grandmother dead from an overdose of sleeping pills. My grandfather, who was like my brother, died when I was twenty-four; my father died in 1991 and eight months later my best friend and nursing mentor jumped off a twenty-story building. All dead. And now there was a chance I'd incur another loss. My breast. The part of a woman that most signifies her femininity. Part of me was getting ready to die.

How do I know I won't die on the operating room table? When I was a nursing student back in 1980, I watched a young man die during open-heart surgery. It was awful. They said he had an excellent chance of success, but something went wrong. Everyone was surprised. I suppose they'll tell my family the same thing. "She's young and in good health, and can withstand the surgery." What about my psyche? Can it survive the surgery? I've always been so concerned with my looks. I work out three times a week and my grandfather taught me to dress nice, even if I only went to the mailbox to mail a letter.

"Hello, this is Dr. Silverstein, is your husband there?"

"Hold on, do you mind being on the speaker phone?"

"Not at all."

"Hi, Dr. Silverstein, Simon here."

"Hi, Simon. I'm glad you're home. Well, there's good news and bad news. The good news is that whatever we found was early and the bad news," he added without even taking a breath, "is that DCIS is quite diffuse around the breast."

Although I was right beside the phone, I slipped out of the moment. My physical body remained on the sofa, yet my mind slid out the window towards the bamboo tree outside my home office window. Denial over-powered me.

"As I explained to Diana when she was here," he continued, "DCIS means small cancer cells have begun to settle and grow in the mammary ducts. As far as I know there is only slight micro-invasion, but how extensive it is, I won't know until surgery."

Although we sat beside one another, I only heard fragments of the remainder of the conversation; his dialogue became blurred, as I doodled, and Simon took copious mental notes.

My eyes reached back outdoors, as if the bamboo tree would console me or offer some clues. I looked beyond the blue sky sprinkled with clouds as the sun began setting in the horizon. I had never prayed, but I instinctively looked up into the heavens and pleaded with my father to make everything right.

My focus returned to my office, and then tossed back into the eyes of my lover, my husband of twenty-four years, and the black and white school photos of the three kids hanging on the office wall. The innocence in their eyes made me tear. I just couldn't focus on the doctor's words, all I kept thinking was, "This must be a mistake."

Half an hour later we thanked Dr. Silverstein and both sat on the golden black velour sofa in the office. Simon drew me close, holding me as tight as he had the day my father died. I felt soothed by the pain of his strong arms. We were silent for five minutes until he blurted out, "Fuck." We looked at each other and banged foreheads as if the notion would make the news sink in, or falsify it.

I wanted to be dead. I thought that would be a good alternative to mutilating the part of me that had nursed and nurtured my three children. The part of me men glance at when not noticing my eyes first.

Still sitting on the sofa, Simon caressed both my breasts. I became more aware of them than ever before. I felt every throb, every tingle, and every squeeze. I wanted to flood my memory with those feelings. Instantly, I felt thankful for all the years that I was bestowed with two perfect breasts. My senses were heightened. I listened to every compliment and each reminder of my beauty as a woman. I soaked up every comment like a sponge; I couldn't get enough reinforcement.

I wanted to be like Gilda Radner from Saturday Night Live and have a sense of humor about what was happening to me. I reread her book, *It's Always Something*, where she spoke about her experience with ovarian cancer. Her introduction read like this:

> Cancer is probably the most unfunny thing in the world, but I'm a comedienne, and even cancer couldn't stop me from seeing humor in what I went through. So I'm sharing with you what I call a seriously funny book, one that confirms my father's favorite expression about life. "It's always something." Although it helped lighten things up for me, it didn't cancel out the truth about me having cancer.

My daughter Regine, had the best comment, though, while trying to console me after she heard the news. "Mom, I see a book here." She reminisced about how I wrote a book in the eighties (which is still in print) about difficult pregnancies, after enduring three of them myself. Looking at the lighter or positive side of things can only help the psyche. I appreciated her comment and filed it away in the archives of my mind, perhaps to be excavated at a later ate, like now, nearly two years later as I set out to write a book about my experience.

Dr. Silverstein recommended a mastectomy and reconstruction. A small two-centimeter area had broken out of the ducts and became invasive. "If I remove all of the calcified areas, your breast will be severely deformed, plus you'll need chemotherapy and radiation. It's your choice, but if you were my wife, I'd chose the former."

How can you argue with that? I opted for a mastectomy and reconstruction.

I deeply trusted Dr. Silverstein and decided to return to L.A. for the surgery. I was put in contact with Dr. Randolph Sherman, the plastic surgeon with whom Dr. Silverstein worked most closely. We had ongoing phone discussions to ascertain the best type of reconstruction for me. After days of agonizing over the decision, and speaking to people at *Women's Information Network Against Breast Cancer* and others who'd endured the surgeries, I opted for the latismis dorsi flap (removal of a muscle from my back to cup the implant). Although the expander was more appealing and involved less surgery and a scar-free back, it was not an option; I couldn't find a local surgeon to perform the weekly inflations.

The next two weeks were like an emotional roller coaster. Simon's parents agreed to stay at our house with the kids while we headed to California for two weeks.

Even my experience as a nurse couldn't prepare me for this surgery. I'd had three cesareans, a menisectomy (knee surgery), and a tonsillectomy, but never in my life had I experienced anything like this. I felt mutilated and robbed of all my womanhood. I couldn't stand looking in the mirror at the body that had borne three magnificent children. It took me days to even glance down at my breasts, something I insisted on doing for the first time with Dr. Sherman. The postoperative period was grueling, laden with pain, discomfort, and tears. The mastectomy site was numb; most of the pain came from my back.

Well, that was then, and now is now. One and a half years later. I feel great and won't let anyone get me down. I frown while reading reports as to the causes of breast cancer. They misled me and are misleading millions of Americans. I did everything necessary to minimize my risks. I believe that we are dealt a card at birth and our life goes according to that card. We are what we are. I have no other answers.

Having the support of my wonderful husband who stayed by my side every inch of the way was what pulled me through and made me the strong woman I am today. Being diagnosed with breast cancer was a life-changing event. The scare taught me the value of life, forced me to slow down and smell the roses a bit more. I've begun yoga and I am writing and reading voraciously. At the age of forty-eight, I've gone back for my M.F.A. in Writing and have a new lease on life. People tell me I look better than ever, and I feel it too. I am a survivor. I am lucky.

In the White Rooms

By Sarah Sutro

After I'd been diagnosed with breast cancer, like many patients, I was delivered to room after room to visit various doctors. I was in a state of disbelief, with the thoughts endlessly revolving in my mind. How did this happen? How could this have happened? Now what is going to happen? Presented with many white appointment cards, I would show up at the appropriate day and time and be taken to one of these white rooms—clearly not anyone's room: no pictures of family or evidence of settling in. No papers or books to speak of, no hangings or bits of clothing or decorative clocks. Usually a low-key, generic bit of art on the walls: a print, a pastel landscape, or a still life.

After being ushered into the room I would take a seat, and eventually the doctor I was supposed to see would show up: the head oncologist or regular oncologist or surgeon. I would sit in all the whiteness, feeling suspended.

The first time the doctor had arrived before me—after the early morning phone call, after I already knew the diagnosis. I came with a friend, as my husband was out of town, and found the surgeon sitting behind an anonymous desk, waiting to draw diagrams and answer questions.

But, usually, I sat in one of these rooms for a few minutes by myself until someone came. My agitated, high velocity thoughts contrasted with the cool, quiet, soulless interior of the room. The building had large windows (the breast center was on the third floor) so the glimpse I had of the outside was also minimal, treetops and a lot of sky.

At times I felt as if I were in some sort of airport, being shunted from waiting room to waiting room. The anonymity of airports, their lack of specificity and their use, over time, by so many people, all headed in the same direction—out. A surreal airport, since I had not chosen or volunteered to go on this trip. And where was I going? It seemed possible, in those early hours and days and weeks, that the destination on my ticket was marked: UNKNOWN, and for all I knew it was a one-way ticket and could end in death.

I was processed through these new airport-like spaces, given this ticket through the white rooms by my initial diagnosis of infiltrating carcinoma. No alternate route or exit, or another flight to choose from. Given the right books, the right instructions, and the white cards, leading to the white rooms.

I look back at that time in wonder. How did I keep myself from falling apart in the enormous white spaces that extended from those white rooms? The mind has an infinite capacity to embroider and invent, and mine did, freely, during those first weeks. My mind tried to tie together loose ends that had happened in the last 47 years that might point to this experience. Like a bad novelist, it projected a tragic outcome because I had watched a morose film in junior high called *Dark Victory*, in which a woman dying of a brain tumor managed to hide it from her husband to spare him her last, dying hour. It wove a dire ending out of a story I wrote in 1st grade about a flower dying because the medicine the other flowers gave it didn't work. Like a computer my mind ransacked the files of my life and thoughts, looking for clues, trying to tie the story line together. What did it mean that I had thought, in my late twenties—like most of my generation, bred on artistic myths of young genius—that I would die young? Why had I never been able to imagine how I would be when I was old? These thought tormented me as I tried to sleep through the first nights of awareness, and as I lived through days of waiting to have the surgery I elected, then the one I was directed toward.

In the first white office room, where my surgeon sat waiting to explain the diagnosis I'd heard only hours earlier, I watched as he drew a picture of cancer, the ducts, the lobes, the infiltration, and filled the paper with options, arrows and a sequence that moved, in terms of treatment, from moderate to severe.

There was lumpectomy, often assumed to be adequate, which preserved so much of the breast that no plastic surgery would be needed or offered. An arrow from lumpectomy pointed to radiation, which often accompanied it: a finishing off of the bad cells that might be left at the site. Another arrow led further down and to the right, almost touching the corner (and therefore, it seemed, remote and unlikely), mastectomy, and, as if an afterthought, chemotherapy and reconstruction.

Most of these terms were new to me, and, in my emotional nightmare state, I could only seem to take in the first part of this treatment roadmap. Did it only seem to me that we focused on lumpectomy as if the rest were only a distant unlikely possibility? My eyes stayed resolutely on the center of the drawing, barely recording the other long terms that hovered dangerously, but remotely in the south-south-east corner of this new, charged territory.

I had a lumpectomy, but as I was to discover four days later, the breast tissue, after wide excision, had to be analyzed at the pathology department of the hospital. Nodes were removed that day, although at that point I didn't even know what nodes were. Several days later the nurse called me, excited, to say she had wonderful news—the nodes were all negative. There was no spread of the disease.

But when my husband and I went in for the post-op appointment, we were invited into another white room where the surgeon explained that the margins of the excision were involved extensively with in situ cancer. He pushed a paper towards us on which he'd written the word MASECTOMY.

We stumbled home in disbelief (this wasn't supposed to happen to us, or anyone else) and then waited four weeks, equivocating about reconstruction, and visiting more white rooms, where we learned statistics about the benefits of chemotherapy and where ratios of menopausal to pre-menopausal symptoms left dangling questions in the air I didn't know how to answer.

In the end, I moved to the south-south-east corner of that original map, undergoing mastectomy, reconstruction, and then six months of chemotherapy. The white rooms of the chemo center were less impersonal than the original office rooms, mainly because there were other people in them, also undergoing treatment, and we could talk, and be there with each other. There were even friends whom I knew from cancer support groups that had formed when I was in early treatment, also having treatment.

I survived the white rooms. I got well and stayed well. The ticket I'd been handed, stamped MAYBE, and DESTINATION UNKNOWN still works as a return, although with no guarantee. But I have a new, sharp appreciation of those one-way circumstances many of us find ourselves in, when choice is pretty much thrown out the window, and we're embarking on a journey like an astronaut another century from now, but with no luggage or map of the territory. And of those wide-open spaces created by the mind, leading from those white rooms—so bare, so impersonal, so uncertain.

Palliative

by Ruthann Robson

I don't believe I knew this term. Recently, the precision of my vocabulary, if nothing else, is improving. Sarcoma (a cancer arising in the connective tissue); retroperitoneal (outside the abdominal organs); metastasis (the movement of malignancy from one part of the body to another); hepatic (pertaining to the liver). Words derived from the Greek (-oma: tumor; retro-: backward; meta-: change). Palliative, from the dead language of Latin, palliatus: cloaked; to alleviate or relieve, but not to cure.

I don't believe that I am using an old Taber's Cyclopedic Medical Dictionary to decipher my body, to salvage it. The book remains a small rectangle of green, though everything else has become shapeless and colorless. It couldn't have been that long ago that I used Taber's to translate the Greco and Latinate labels in the reports from government doctors. Government doctors who concluded my clients—former-farmworkers, former-domestics, former-day-laborers—were able to continue working. Never mind the missing arms, sight, legs, or the mental stability to set an alarm clock. Poverty, an entry in Taber's, between Poupert's ligament and povidine iodine, was not included in the government doctors' terminology.

I don't believe the way the doctors at the famous cancer center speak to me. Their cadences are sharp, harsh, dismissive. I suppose they are careless, jaded, at home in a language they use to talk to those who will soon be homeless, in that most ultimate sense. When I ask a question, a bit of Greek or Latin is volleyed back, often with the footnote: That is, if you really need to know the precise name.

The unsaid: No appellation will assist you. I ask for the spelling any-way. I take careful notes. I consult Taber's. As if biopsies and CT scans are tests for which one can prepare.

I don't believe it is the surgeon's secretary who telephones to tell me the result of the liver biopsy: radio suspicious. This is not in Taber's, but I know it means hopeless. I ask for the report. It is two lines, no sentences. One of which is what the secretary stated. The other of which is well-differentiated cells. This is not in Taber's dictionary either. But well cannot mean well; well must mean very, and for the cancer cells to be very different from the ordinary cells confirms that it is hopeless. The surgeon's secretary tells me that no surgery is indicated: it would only be palliative.

I don't believe phrases can sound so dissonant. How palliative, well-differentiated, radio suspicious, assume a different melody in the mouths of those at the not-so-famous cancer center. People live with incurable diseases for years, the oncologist sings a hymn to diabetes, a disease that is chronic (from the Greek, chronos: time). There's nothing wrong with palliative, the surgeon hums, before his incisions score my retroperi-toneum. The more different the cancer cells from the ordinary cells, the better, I learn from a nurse whose husband will soon die from the same disease, his cancer cells being not so well-differentiated. Your suspicious liver has been vindicated, the radiologist delivers his verdict in a one-word aria: hemangioma. Notes from the libretto: from the Greek, that living language (haima: blood; angeion: vessel; -oma: tumor), meaning a benign tumor of dilated blood vessels. Benign (from the Latin, mild): the opposite of malignant; not recurrent or progressive.

I don't believe in language, in doctors, or that tragedy can transmute into a comedy. Of errors, misdiagnosis, malpractice. And then I do. In fragments, unfunny and unfocused. Humor (from the Latin, fluid) eludes me. Comedy (from the Greek, revel, or from the Latin, village) "begins in harshness and ends happily," at least according to Dante, who navigates from the Inferno to Paradise without ever resorting to Taber's Cyclopedic Medical Dictionary.

I can't believe I'm alive (from the Old English, meaning that I will be old, meaning that I might travel to England or to Greece, meaning that I can speak with a tongue coated in dictionaries, meaning that I am relieved to wear that dark and dirty cloak called time, however frayed by uncertainty.)

Contributors Notes

Ruthann Robson is on the board of www.sairorna.net, a Website devoted to the rare cancer of sarcoma, with which she was diagnosed in 1998 and from which she is now in remission. She is a professor of law at the City University of New York School of Law and has written widely on lesbian legal theory, including *Sappho Goes to Law School* (Columbia Univ. Press 1998). She also is the author of several novels, including *A/K/A* (St. Martin's Press 1998).

Judith Boothby has practiced chiropractic for sixteen years. In 1996 she received the "Young Chiropractor Of The Year" award from the CAO. She has a master's degree from MIT and has helped develop radiation therapy computer software for Massachusetts General Hospital. She lives in Portland, Oregon with her teenage son.

Milton Ricketts, age 75, is a retired engineer who worked for Bell System before becoming an independent consultant in the US, Eastern Europe, and Southeast Asia. He and his wife Carol have enjoyed sailboat racing as well as coastal and offshore cruising for over 57 years. Both are dedicated physical fitness advocates.

Deborah Derrickson Kossmann, Psy.D. is a licensed clinical psychologist in private practice in Langhorne, PA outside of Philadelphia. Her specialties include trauma, grief, and health psychology. When this essay was written, she was also working part time in a multidisciplinary medical oncology practice. She is a journalist, essayist, and poet.

Bara Swain is the recipient of a dozen writing grants for plays and prose. Recent accomplishments: *His Unjust Dessert,* essay; *Love is Ageless: Stories About Alzheimer's Disease*; "Your Health Comes First … You Can Always Hang Yourself Later," a dramatic reading of selected stories (Kaufman Theater, American Museum of Natural History); "The Daughter," short story, *Long Shot Magazine*, and "Pull," finalist, Lamia Ink! International One-Page Play Festival (NYC). She is currently working on a collection of nine monologues, entitled *ICD-9*. Her writing is inspired by the spirit of her deceased husband and renewed by the spirit of their 16-year-old daughter.

David Ross is a licensed clinical social worker and psychotherapist living in San Diego, CA. His passion is helping others use limitation and illness to transform and empower their lives toward deeper meaning and wisdom. He is a motivational speaker, seminar leader, and mentor and can be reached at 619-297-4211 or via e-mail at rossdm@prodigy.net.

Kathryn Kerr is an adjunct English professor at Illinois State University.

Diana Marquise Raab has been a writer for more than twenty-eight years. As a registered nurse, she wrote and self-published *Getting Pregnant and Staying Pregnant: A guide to high-risk pregnancy* in 1985. In 1987, the book right were sold to Hunter House Publishers (California) and is now in its third edition. In 1992, the book won the PMA's Benjamin Franklin Book Award for best health and wellness book. "Lucknow Woman" recently won honorable mention in The Metrouniversity Writing Competition for Graduate Students.

Sarah Sutro is an artist and writer recently returned from living and working in Bangladesh. She was worked in the Fogg and Johnson Museums. Recipient of a Pollock Krasner Grant and MacDowell fellowships, she has taught at Emerson College, Lesley University, and the Museum School. Her work is at www.sarahsutro.com.